Y0-BZA-391

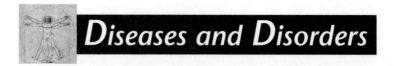
Diseases and Disorders

Lyme
Disease

Titles in the Diseases and Disorders series include:

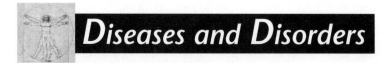
Diseases and Disorders

Lyme Disease

by Gail B. Stewart

LUCENT BOOKS®

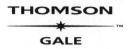

THOMSON
™
GALE

San Diego • Detroit • New York • San Francisco • Cleveland
New Haven, Conn. • Waterville, Maine • London • Munich

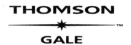

© 2003 by Lucent Books. Lucent Books is an imprint of The Gale Group, Inc.,
a division of Thomson Learning, Inc.

Lucent Books® and Thomson Learning™ are trademarks used herein under license.

For more information, contact
Lucent Books
27500 Drake Rd.
Farmington Hills, MI 48331-3535
Or you can visit our Internet site at http://www.gale.com

LIBRARY OF CONGRESS CATALOGING-IN-PUBLICATION DATA

Stewart, Gail B., 1949–
    Lyme disease / by Gail B. Stewart.
p. cm. — (Diseases and disorders)
Summary: Discusses the history, symptoms, diagnosis, and treatment of Lyme disease,
current research into cures, and the challenges of living with the disease.
Includes bibliographical references and index.
    ISBN 1-56006-907-4 (hbk. : alk. paper)
    1. Lyme disease—Juvenile literature. [1. Lyme disease. 2. Diseases.] I. Title. II. Diseases
and disorders series.
    RC155.5 .S74 2004
    616.9'2—dc21

                                                          2002153400

Printed in the United States of America

Table of Contents

"The Most Difficult Puzzles Ever Devised"

C HARLES BEST, ONE of the pioneers in the search for a cure for
diabetes, once explained what it is about medical research
that intrigued him so. "It's not just the gratification of knowing
one is helping people," he confided, "although that probably is a
more heroic and selfless motivation. Those feelings may enter in,
but truly, what I find best is the feeling of going toe to toe with
nature, of trying to solve the most difficult puzzles ever devised.
The answers are there somewhere, those keys that will solve the
puzzle and make the patient well. But how will those keys be
found?"

Since the dawn of civilization, nothing has so puzzled people—
and often frightened them, as well—as the onset of illness in a
body or mind that had seemed healthy before. A seizure, the inability of a heart to pump, the sudden deterioration of muscle
tone in a small child—being unable to reverse such conditions or
even to understand why they occur was unspeakably frustrating
to healers. Even before there were names for such conditions,
even before they were understood at all, each was a reminder of
how complex the human body was, and how vulnerable.

While our grappling with understanding diseases has been
frustrating at times, it has also provided some of humankind's
most heroic accomplishments. Alexander Fleming's accidental
discovery in 1928 of a mold that could be turned into penicillin

has resulted in the saving of untold millions of lives. The isolation of the enzyme insulin has reversed what was once a death sentence for anyone with diabetes. There have been great strides in combating conditions for which there is not yet a cure, too. Medicines can help AIDS patients live longer, diagnostic tools such as mammography and ultrasounds can help doctors find tumors while they are treatable, and laser surgery techniques have made the most intricate, minute operations routine.

This "toe-to-toe" competition with diseases and disorders is even more remarkable when seen in a historical continuum. An astonishing amount of progress has been made in a very short time. Just two hundred years ago, the existence of germs as a cause of some diseases was unknown. In fact, it was less than 150 years ago that a British surgeon named Joseph Lister had difficulty persuading his fellow doctors that washing their hands before delivering a baby might increase the chances of a healthy delivery (especially if they had just attended to a diseased patient)!

Each book in Lucent's Diseases and Disorders series explores a disease or disorder and the knowledge that has been accumulated (or discarded) by doctors through the years. Each book also examines the tools used for pinpointing a diagnosis, as well as the various means that are used to treat or cure a disease. Finally, new ideas are presented—techniques or medicines that may be on the horizon.

Frustration and disappointment are still part of medicine, for not every disease or condition can be cured or prevented. But the limitations of knowledge are being pushed outward constantly; the "most difficult puzzles ever devised" are finding challengers every day.

The Faces of Lyme Disease

It should have been an exciting time for Chelsea. At eighteen, she was busy getting ready to start her first year of college. For the past month, she and her parents had been carefully assembling all of the clothes, school supplies, and other essentials she would need to start her life as a college freshman. But on August 30, the day before she was due to leave for college, Chelsea began having pains in her right knee.

"It Was the Size of Two Knees"

At first Chelsea thought maybe she had hurt it when she was shooting baskets outside with a neighbor a few days earlier.

"I figured I twisted it without realizing it or something," she said. "I mean, I don't remember ever hurting it, but I tried to look at it logically. I just decided to stay off it, and I hung around the house watching TV and stuff. I put ice on it, and by that night, I thought maybe it was feeling a little better.

"But the next day I was worse," she said. "My knee was so swollen—it was the size of two knees! I had a very red rash on the side of my knee, too, which I hadn't had at first. Anyway, I was really scared. My mom took me in to the doctor and they x-rayed it, but didn't find anything. But while I was talking to the nurse, I mentioned I'd been working as a camp counselor in Wisconsin a couple months earlier. And because there are ticks in the woods where the camp was, they decided to do a blood test for Lyme disease. And that's exactly what I had—the test came back positive."

Chelsea was put on strong antibiotics—first for three days in the hospital where the doctor could regulate the dose—and then for four weeks afterward. She needed crutches to walk.

"It took a couple of months, really, before my knee was completely back to normal," she remembers. "And I was really late starting school—I missed freshman orientation and everything, so I was two steps behind everyone else for a little while. I had to take the pills for almost four weeks, but it was so great feeling healthy again. I still think about it, how odd it was that I had such a serious disease from a tick—that I don't even remember biting me."[1]

Two Hundred Ticks

While Chelsea could not remember being bitten by a tick, professional golfer Tim Simpson has a very vivid memory of his own tick bites. Hunting with a friend in 1991, he awoke one morning in his cabin to find about two hundred ticks covering his chest. A week later, he was very ill with what felt like a bad case of the flu.

Infected tick nymphs of the genus Ixodes *transmit bacteria that cause Lyme disease.*

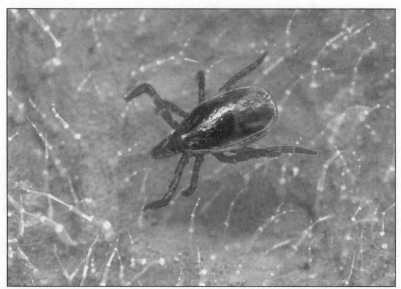

As *USA Today* later reported, the thirty-four-year-old golfer "had constant fevers; he was so weak he couldn't pick up his thirty-pound daughter. He had to lie in bed at night with ice packs on his joints to fight the arthritic pain. He had headaches, swollen glands, sweats, and fatigue."[2]

He was diagnosed with Lyme disease, and although doctors wanted to hospitalize him, Simpson opted instead to stay on the PGA Tour and take medicine on his own. After all, he was earning a great deal of money; at the top of his game just before being struck with Lyme disease, he had even been a contender for the prestigious Ryder Cup team.

Ridicule

But it was soon evident that the disease was far stronger than Simpson. He could handle the loss of strength and energy, but the constant shaking of his hands made golf impossible. "Simpson's hands shook so badly," wrote one reporter, "that when he stood over the ball, if he wasn't careful, he would knock a two-foot putt 25 feet past the cup and into a sand trap."[3]

Golf experts, who knew nothing about his illness, speculated that he had peaked and was simply in decline. As he missed the qualifying cuts for tournament after tournament, he was glibly written off as one of the "Flops of '91" by a national golf magzine. Finally, after struggling to walk the eighteen holes of the first round of the Greensboro Open in April 1992, Simpson walked away from the game.

He vowed to return after he felt better. In November 1996, he was still feeling some of the effects of Lyme disease, though he did not want to rule out a comeback. "If my hands ever stop shaking," he told reporters, "I'll get back to the top."[4]

David's Lyme Disease

David (not his real name) has battled the effects of Lyme disease for almost seventeen years. Like Chelsea, he had a rash and swollen knees. He also suffered from fatigue and aching muscles. In 1984, doctors told him it was a virus, and it would go away on its own.

"They just said to lie low," he said, "and it would go away on its own. They said that because it was viral rather than bacterial, and that penicillin and stuff like that wouldn't do any good. So I did. And it finally did get better for a week, maybe. Then it came back.

"See, the symptoms kept changing. Sometimes it was the feeling of having the flu. Then it was my knees, and the glands on my neck that were swollen. Then I got a really severe eye infection, and the right side of my face was numb. About a month after that I started having trouble walking."

Anger and Depression

The doctor changed his diagnosis from a virus to arthritis, said David. But when he started having trouble remembering things and expressing himself, he was told he had MS—multiple sclerosis. Confused and frustrated, he found it difficult to continue his job as a landscaper.

"I couldn't do anything," he said. "I was so down, so depressed. I felt like the doctor didn't have a clue, and at the same time, that nobody over [at the clinic] even cared. I felt like they thought I was making up symptoms. But I wasn't. And my health was getting worse and worse."

David said that it was not until almost two years had gone by after his first doctor's appointment that anyone suggested Lyme disease as a cause for his problems.

"I had two Lyme tests," he said. "The results showed I had it, and a real high number of the Lyme germs, too. Way more than a lot of the people with Lyme. But they [the doctors] haven't been able to make it go away. It's in my brain and my heart and just about every other place in my body. I can't walk more than a few steps before I get chest pains, you know, from my heart. And even if my heart didn't hurt, my legs wouldn't let me go much more than that, anyway. I still am prone to eye infections and swollen glands and fevers just spiking out of the blue. It's a bad way to live."[5]

"We Have Wasted Valuable Time"

Although their symptoms vary widely, these three people were all victims of Lyme disease, an illness that has become extremely common in the United States. In September 2002, the Lyme Disease Foundation, which is a clearinghouse for information and public awareness, declared Lyme disease one of the fastest-growing infectious diseases in the United States. Since 1980, more than 193,000 cases have been reported in the United States. In 2000, there were 17,730 documented cases of Lyme disease—an increase of 8 percent from 1999.

However, many infectious disease experts feel that the actual number of cases could be ten times that—as many as 1.9 million in the past twenty-one years. This is due to the fact that, unlike most illnesses, which are routinely diagnosed by doctors on the basis of a set of common symptoms, Lyme disease has proved to be extremely difficult to identify. Many scientists call Lyme disease "the great imitator" because of its frustrating tendency to take on the symptoms of other diseases.

For that reason, Lyme disease has been a source of confusion and frustration for doctors. "We have the ability to cure [Lyme disease] easily with antibiotics if we can diagnose it fairly quickly," says one health professional. "But too often, especially in the past, we have wasted valuable time by assuming it's something else."[6]

As frustrating as Lyme disease may be for doctors, it is far more so for patients. "Having a disease that doctors don't always recognize can be scary," says the mother of one Lyme disease patient. "You feel like you want answers just as much as you want relief. And lots of people with Lyme disease don't get either one very quickly."[7]

This tick-transmitted disease, which can have dozens of symptoms that may not occur for months after the bite, has proved to be a nightmare for both doctors and patients. The one aspect of Lyme disease that is clear is that when caught early, it almost always can be easily cured. And the more one knows about the disease, the ticks that spread it, and the symptoms of Lyme disease, the better one's chances of avoiding it entirely.

Chapter 1

The Sickness Without a Name

Though it has been getting a great deal of attention in recent years, Lyme disease is not new. People have been getting sick from the bacteria that cause the illness for many years. However, until 1975, scientists had not identified the bacteria or named the disease. Because Lyme disease has symptoms that seem like those of other well-known diseases, doctors made assumptions that were not true.

Cancer? Arthritis? Alzheimer's Disease?

Some people with Lyme disease were thought to have a bad case of the flu. Others, who experienced swelling and stiffness, were told that they had arthritis or multiple sclerosis. Still others who experienced heart or nervous system trouble were diagnosed with everything from cancer to chronic fatigue syndrome, from Alzheimer's disease to congenital heart failure. Some were simply dismissed by their doctors as being so hysterical and nervous about their health that they were making themselves sick.

Not surprisingly, those patients who were misdiagnosed were not given the proper treatment. They might improve for a time on certain medications, but after a week or two, their symptoms would return—and sometimes they would be more severe than before. As a result, these patients became progressively sicker—and definitely more frustrated.

One town in Connecticut, called Lyme, was seeing a great many chronic illnesses that seemed to have doctors stumped in the mid-1970s. In fact, it was largely because of the efforts of a

Lyme resident named Polly Murray that state medical authorities first learned of the scope of the problem.

"My Legs Would Start Twitching and Jerking Uncontrollably"

Murray, an artist and mother of four children, had struggled for years with a variety of health problems. She had high fevers and swollen joints. She got sore throats and severe rashes that could not be explained. Large black-and-blue marks—unrelated to bruises or bumps—erupted on her legs. She suffered from bone-numbing fatigue and headaches, too. The symptoms seemed unrelated to one another, so her doctors treated each as if it were a separate problem. She was often given antibiotics, which would seem to help for a little while. But always, once she was through with her prescribed medicine, another health problem would arise.

Murray later wrote of the suddenness and severity of some of the problems she experienced. "I would get sudden headaches, so excruciatingly painful that I would want to close my eyes and sleep," she recalls. "The bouts of sore throats and laryngitis continued. I had

Skin rashes associated with Lyme disease often appear as rose-colored bull's-eye shapes and range from two to fourteen inches in diameter.

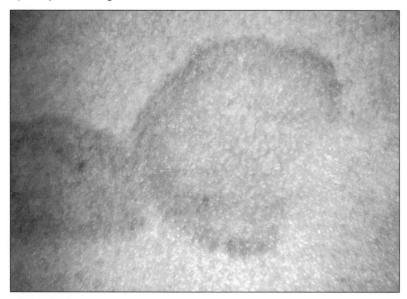

periodic shooting pains in my legs, hips, and knees. At times, my knee felt as if it were popping out of joint."[8]

As the months went on, her symptoms became almost continuous. "In December [1970]," she writes, "my neck and shoulder became stiff and painful, making driving and moving around almost impossible. I could hardly lift my left arm. It hurt to turn over in bed, and if I woke up in the night, my legs would start twitching and jerking uncontrollably, making getting back to sleep difficult. It was frustrating just finding a comfortable position."[9]

"What Is the Matter with Me?"

Even more frustrating for Murray was finding the source of her problems. She had always been healthy, but in the early 1970s she could hardly get through a week without calling the doctor. Although her doctors were sympathetic at first, they grew impatient when she requested second opinions on their diagnoses. One scolded her for her persistence, saying, "Please, please, accept the fact that everything has been done and forget this fruitless search for a label [for your symptoms]. We can do no more."[10]

She insisted, however, and spent weeks at a time in various hospitals, undergoing scores of tests and evaluations. When one doctor suggested that perhaps she *wanted* to be sick—that her illnesses were more psychological than physical—she willingly submitted to psychiatric evaluations, too. But these provided doctors with no more answers than the medical tests had.

The constant illness, together with the lack of understanding and help from doctors, was understandably depressing. "I was so tired in those days," Murray says, "so tired of asking, 'What is the matter with me?' only to be told again and again that my symptoms fit no known disease."[11]

Intensifying the Search

It is difficult to know what would have happened to Murray's resolve to find the reason for her poor health if she remained the only one in her family that was sick. But by 1975, her entire family was experiencing numerous symptoms, too. Two were on crutches because of painfully swollen knees, although neither could remember hurting themselves. Others had insomnia, ringing in their ears, nosebleeds, and swollen joints. And all seemed to have experienced a bull's-eye-shaped rash at one time or another. Even the family dog was sick—she had trouble walking and had uncontrollable twitching in her legs at times.

Frightened for her family, Murray began keeping a journal of each symptom she, her husband, or their children experienced. She wrote what the doctor's diagnosis was, and what, if any, medicines were prescribed. She continued to talk to doctors about the mysterious illnesses, but she also began to talk with other mothers in Lyme.

In doing so, she learned that many of them had experienced—or knew someone else who had experienced—some of the same symptoms the Murrays had. "Once I started asking questions," Murray wrote, "I found that there were quite a few with almost the same story, although not with as many victims within the same family."[12] In fact, in the months ahead, Murray found thirty-five cases in Lyme that seemed to have the same symptoms as the ones she and her family had experienced. The Murrays, it seemed, were not the only ones with this disease. But what was it?

Too Much JRA

One of the most frequent symptoms, besides the rash, was the swelling and stiffness of joints—especially the knees and ankles. This is a common symptom of arthritis, a disease that is common in older people. There is a form of the disease called juvenile rheumatoid arthritis, or JRA, which can affect children. In fact, doctors had diagnosed two of Murray's sons as having the disease. But the more Murray read about JRA, the more dissatisfied she was with the doctors' diagnoses. JRA was considered quite rare—affecting only one in 100,000 children—and was not contagious. Was it not odd that she had two sons with the disease, and that neighbors she talked to had the same symptoms?

In October 1975, Murray decided to call the Connecticut Health Department with her concerns. State medical workers keep statistics on outbreaks of certain diseases. She briefly told

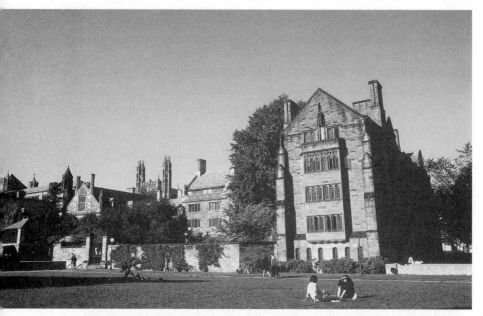

Polly Murray was referred to a doctor at Yale University (pictured) after several physicians were unable to pinpoint the source of her ailments.

them about the symptoms her family and others had been experiencing. She asked if they knew of any virus that had arthritis-like symptoms that could be causing the problems in Lyme.

Officials knew of no such outbreak but urged her to call Dr. Allen Steere, an arthritis specialist at Yale University. Steere was immediately interested and agreed to study the problem of what could be causing so much JRA (or something that had symptoms like it) in a town as small as Lyme.

Investigating "Lyme Arthritis"

At first, Steere and his colleagues collected as much information as they could about the people who were sick. They asked dozens of questions, trying to pinpoint how, where, and when each person became sick. They also contacted doctors in the area, asking them to be on the alert for symptoms of this mysterious ailment. Since Murray and her family were still being plagued by various symptoms, Steere asked her to document swollen joints and rashes by taking photographs when possible.

This documentation would help doctors understand the range of symptoms to watch for.

After almost six months, the study had identified thirty-nine children and twelve adults who lived in or near Lyme and had symptoms of arthritis. At this point, Steere assumed this illness was indeed a form of arthritis, as is evident in a letter he sent to the residents of Lyme in May 1976:

> After six months, we have finished the first phase of our study of patients with "Lyme arthritis" . . . . It is characterized by usually short and mild but often recurrent attacks of pain and swelling in a relatively few large joints, especially the knees, with longer intervening periods of no symptoms at all. No patients have had permanent injury to joints. . . . The best treatment for the usually mild symptoms of arthritis is not yet clear. At present we suggest taking only aspirin.[13]

Though Murray and others had indicated to the researchers that they had suffered more symptoms than just the rash and swollen joints, Steere and his colleagues were not convinced at first that the other symptoms were related. Over the next several months, however, the evidence seemed to indicate this was, in fact, much more than a new form of arthritis. There were so many cases of severe headaches, nausea, fevers, extreme fatigue, eye problems, irregular heart rhythms, and chronic muscle pain associated with the swollen joints that doctors amended "Lyme arthritis" to "Lyme disease." There was little cause for celebration, however, since identifying a disease was a long way from explaining it.

How Is the Disease Spread?

The research revealed, too, that most of the Lyme residents who had the disease lived near heavily wooded areas, rather than in the center of town. In fact, on some streets in these wooded areas, Steere and his colleagues noted that as many as 10 percent of the children were affected by Lyme disease. The researchers wondered if some sort of insect or spider found in the woods was to blame for spreading the disease.

Early in the summer of 1976 researchers began trapping various animals in the wooded areas around Lyme, inspecting them for parasites and evaluating their health. They set out special traps to attract mosquitoes and other flying insects. They also dragged the lawns and wooded areas, pulling a large piece of white flannel behind them. Many insects, spiders, and ticks stuck to the cloth, and the researchers could inspect them, too.

Ticks, in particular, interested the doctors for a couple of reasons. First, many of the victims of Lyme disease had a skin rash in the weeks or months before they became ill. It was known then that certain tick bites *could* result in rashes. Another aspect of the disease that doctors noted was that it seemed to be seasonal, being far more common in the summer months. That seemed to suggest a virus or other infection that was carried by an insect or a tick.

The most interesting link with ticks as a source of the disease was that Lyme disease was far more common on one side of the Connecticut River, which flows through the middle of the state, than the other side. That was consistent with one particular type of tick collected by researchers. The pinpoint-sized *Ixodes scapularis*,

Dr. Allen Steere and his colleagues realized that cases of people with arthritic symptoms were more common to one side of the Connecticut River (pictured) than the other.

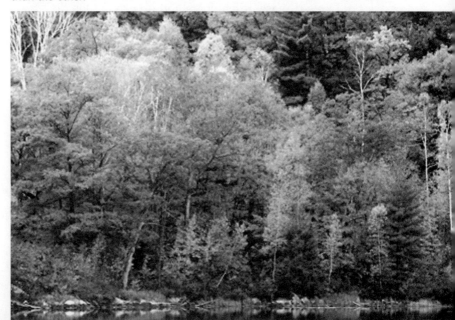

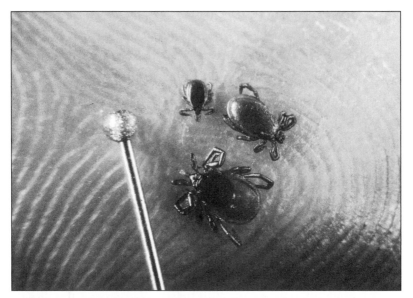

Immature deer ticks barely larger than a pinhead are the most prevalent carriers of spirochetes linked to Lyme disease.

or deer tick, was found in great numbers on the side of the river with the most victims of Lyme disease.

The New Spirochete

Although the data seemed to point to the deer tick as the likely carrier of Lyme disease, researchers had no proof. One doctor explained, "The evidence strongly suggested that Lyme disease was an infectious disease spread by ticks, but the identity of the infections remained a mystery. There are many varieties of ticks, and different ticks carry different agents: viruses, bacteria, protozoa, or even small worms."[14] No one was willing to rule out anything without hard evidence.

It was not until five years later, in 1981, that a scientist in Montana discovered the Lyme disease bacterium—quite by accident. Dr. Willy Burgdorfer had been studying a disease called Rocky Mountain spotted fever, a potentially fatal illness carried by a tiny, one-celled parasite that lives in certain ticks. There had been an outbreak of Rocky Mountain spotted fever on Long Island, in New York. He and his colleagues were dissecting various types of ticks found on Long Island to see how many carried the parasite. He checked several deer ticks, and although he did not find the parasite, he did see something that startled him.

In several of the deer ticks, he found spirochetes—spiral-shaped bacteria that were not ordinarily found in deer ticks. A new type of bacteria found in a tick could be very important, Burgdorfer knew—especially since there was so much talk about the mysterious cause of Lyme disease. On a hunch, he and his assistants checked blood samples of people with Lyme disease. They were excited to see that the blood contained evidence that the patients had been exposed to this spirochete. Subsequent blood tests of other Lyme disease patients confirmed that this spirochete—named *Borrelia burgdorferi*, after the man who discovered it—was the cause of Lyme disease.

The Murrays, like many other residents of Lyme, were astonished when it was finally proved that the cause of their problems had indeed been carried by ticks. Ticks were a fact of life for people who lived in wooded areas like Lyme. Many people shuddered to think of all the ticks they had found on themselves, on their children, and on their pets over the years. Most had not realized that there were different types of ticks. "In those days, a tick was a tick to us," wrote Murray. "We didn't make the distinction between what we know now as dog, wood, and deer ticks. Small ticks were simply thought to be baby ticks."[15]

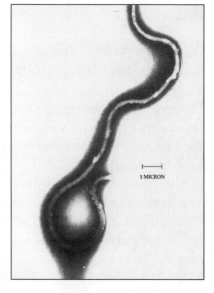

Dr. Willy Burgdorfer discovered the Borrelia burgdorferi *spirochete (pictured).*

I———I
1 MICRON

An Emerging Disease

Interestingly, as the new information was published about the cause of Lyme disease, it became clear that it was not a new disease at all. Instead, it is called an emerging disease—one that was once rare, but has become far more common. In Europe, doctors had known since the early twentieth century about a strange skin rash that they believed began after a person was bitten by an insect or a tick. Over the next several days, the rash moved outward, away from the bite, in a sort of bull's-eye pattern.

Ironically, Dr. B. Lipschutz, an Austrian doctor, quite accurately speculated on the source of the rash in 1902. "Perhaps we are dealing with a skin infection caused through the bite of a tick," he wrote. "Therefore, attention should be directed towards microscopic/bacteriologic investigations of the intestinal tract . . . of the tick."[16] Unfortunately, no one followed through on his idea and dissected the tick to look for such bacteria.

Another reason that American doctors were unaware of the disease's existence was that the European doctors had concentrated on the rash, rather than on the arthritis-like symptoms that sometimes occurred afterward. Because early scientists had not made a link between the rash and other symptoms, they did not imagine that the same bacteria could have caused both. After Burgdorfer's discovery, however, doctors were interested in learning why this fairly rare disease found in Europe in the early twentieth century had begun making Americans ill in increasing numbers.

Spirochetes in DNA

Some speculated at first that the bacteria had been spread to the United States by tick-infested livestock imported from England. However, some remarkable research at several museums proved this theory incorrect. Far from being new to the United States, the bacteria have been here for more than a century—and possibly even longer than that.

The research occurred at several museums, including the Smithsonian Institution in Washington, D.C., and the Museum of Comparative Zoology at Harvard University. These museums had the preserved bodies of several animals, donated in the late nineteenth century by various naturalists. Of particular interest to the Lyme disease researchers were white-footed mice, which

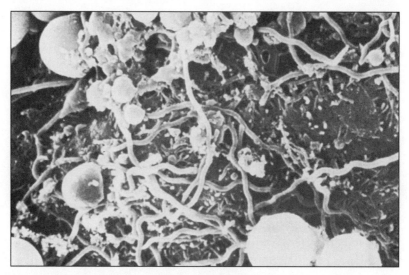

As early as 1902, doctors hypothesized the bacteria leading to Lyme disease existed in the intestinal tract (pictured) of ticks.

were known to carry the deer tick. Using modern DNA-gathering techniques, researchers found traces of *Borrelia burgdorferi* in some of the samples—proving that the bacteria making people sick in the 1970s had been around for a long time.

Having identified the bacterium that causes Lyme disease was extremely important, for it enabled scientists to test the efficiency of various medications in curing the disease. At the same time, researchers knew that there was a great deal left to understand about Lyme disease. They wanted to know why some people bit by the infected deer ticks were unaffected, while some became very ill. And among those with Lyme disease, why were symptoms so different? Finally, they wanted to learn how a tiny spiral-shaped bacterium living in the intestinal tract of a tick the size of a poppy seed could create such problems for human beings.

Chapter 2

From Deer Tick to Human

Most types of bacteria require fairly specific conditions in which to live and reproduce. Some need a certain type of soil or a particular temperature of water. Some live in milk or other dairy products, while some grow best on certain plants. Although many bacteria can adapt to other conditions, most seem to thrive in one specific environment. *Borrelia burgdorferi* (often shortened to Bb) is no different. As one expert explains, there are three important criteria that its environment must meet if the Bb bacterium is to survive:

> First, it needs someplace to live—a host reservoir that has an immune system that does not kill *B. burgdorferi*. Second, in return it must not kill the host, else its life will end, too. Third, since the host is bound to die someday, *B. burgdorferi* needs another host . . . to be a good Samaritan to carry it to another host reservoir so it does not die off with the first one.[17]

Blood is the environment that best suits the Lyme disease bacteria. It is not necessary for the blood to be human. In fact, many kinds of animals can be infected with Bb bacteria—including deer, mice, raccoons, birds, and dogs. The deer tick, coincidentally, also requires the blood of other animals to survive. As it searches for blood, the deer tick becomes the "good Samaritan" that enables the Bb bacteria to get from host to host, so that they can live and reproduce. And it is in looking at the life cycle of this tick that the spread of Lyme disease can best be understood.

"Disgusting Parasitic Animals"

While discovery of a connection between deer ticks and the bacteria causing Lyme disease is a fairly recent one, ticks have long been viewed with derision. Ticks are not insects, but rather belong to the same biological grouping as spiders and mites. As do the other 850 species of ticks on the planet, the deer tick has eight legs and two basic body parts. They do not fly, nor do they have antennae, as insects do. They are considered parasites, which means that they live off the blood of another animal in order to live. Whether because he suspected them of carrying infection or because of the way ticks gorge themselves on blood, the Greek philosopher Aristotle dismissed them as being "disgusting parasitic animals."[18]

Deer ticks live approximately two years. They hatch in the summer from eggs the adult tick lays in the spring. These newly hatched ticks are called larvae. Using the printed page as a reference, scientists say that one deer tick larva is the size of a period. The larvae attach themselves to a mouse, bird, or other small animal and, for the next two days, feed on its blood. After the larvae have drunk their fill, they simply drop off the animal. They will not have to eat again until the following spring.

Raccoons (pictured), deer, dogs, wild rodents, birds, and other animals can contract Borrelia burgdorferi *bacteria.*

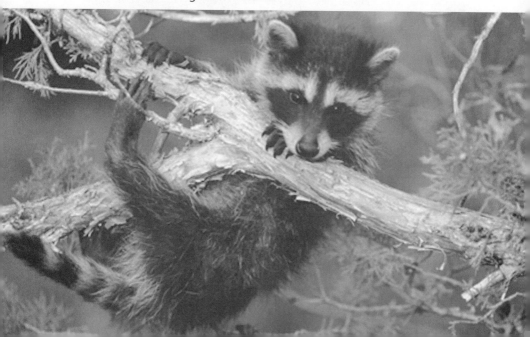

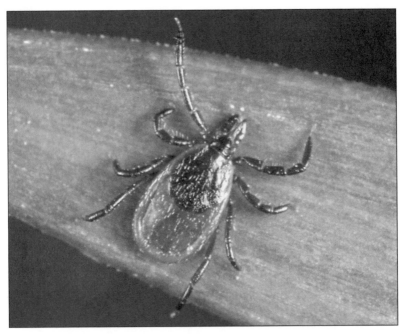

A deer tick (adult female pictured) is actually more closely related to spiders and mites than insects.

After eating that first meal, a larva sheds its outer skeleton and develops a new one. Molting usually takes a few days, after which the larva is called a nymph. Nymphs are larger than larvae—the body (including legs) would fit inside the letter *o*. Like larvae, nymphs instinctively seek a nearby animal and attach themselves to it. After feeding for several days, the nymphs, too, drop off and molt into their new—and final—stage.

A Life of Three Meals

The adult tick is a bit bigger than the nymph; its body, with legs, would fill a capital *O*, although it plumps up to the size of a raisin after feeding. It is as an adult that the deer tick has its third—and last—meal. This final meal lasts between one and two weeks. Immediately before feeding this final time, the ticks mate.

After mating and eating, the males remain on the animal host and eventually die. The females, on the other hand, drop off the host into the leaves on the forest floor. They remain dormant until the following spring, when they lay their eggs—usually between one thousand and three thousand of them. The female dies soon afterward.

Larvae do not hatch hosting Lyme bacteria. As they move through the various stages of their lives, ticks may become infected with the Bb bacteria at any stage—larva, nymph, or adult. They become infected through the blood they feed on—usually from mice, since they are common in the wooded areas in which ticks live.

Sensing a Passing Host

Lacking wings, ticks are not as mobile as many insects. They can crawl, but they do not spend time searching for an animal host. Instead, ticks (larvae, nymphs, and adults) wait for a host to come to them. They usually crawl to the top of a blade of grass or some other vegetation, hang on with their hindmost pair of legs, and reach out with their front legs. This process is called "questing." A special organ on their front legs enables questing ticks to sense the presence of a warm body and carbon dioxide—the gas exhaled by animals as they breathe.

Two-Year Life Cycle of Deer Ticks

Year 1

Spring
Engorged females lay eggs and die.

Summer
Eggs hatch into larvae; larvae eat first meal (from mice, birds).

Fall/Winter
Larvae are dormant.

Year 2

Spring/Summer
Larvae become nymphs; nymphs eat second meal (from mice, deer, small animals, humans).

Fall
Nymphs become adults; adults mate and eat third meal (from mice, deer, small animals, humans).

Winter
Males die; females lie dormant until following spring.

As soon as the tick gets signals that a possible host is passing by, it lets go of the vegetation it is sitting on and attaches itself to the animal. Afterward, it climbs to a spot on the host that is somewhat protected. On a human host, it may settle in hair or in a crease or fold of skin, for example.

Marnie, a woman who had Lyme, felt an itching sensation in the crease of skin behind her knee and was startled to find two deer ticks. "It's not a place that's easy to see, unless you're looking in a full-length mirror," she said. "But I was riding in the car with my husband, and I kept scratching at this spot. I could feel a sort of bump, a raised area behind there. I thought maybe it was a mosquito bite, but it felt too hard. I got curious finally, and I used the mirror in my purse to see what it was. Oh, I was grossed out," she shudders. "I'd never had a tick on me before, and there were two of them, right next to one another."[19]

Kyle, twenty, found a tick while he was shaving. "It was in my beard," he says. "I'd been camping for ten days in Minnesota, and hadn't shaved all that time. . . . I found the tick, completely engorged with blood. I hadn't even felt it, not when it crawled on me, not when it bit me."[20]

After engorging itself on a meal of animal blood, adult female ticks (pictured) usually drop to the forest floor and become dormant until spring.

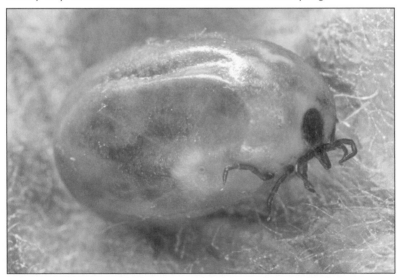

The Chemistry Within a Tick

Once the tick has found a location in which it feels fairly protected, it begins to feed. Because the tick eats so rarely in its life, it must take in almost a year's worth of blood from a single host. To do this, it is crucial for the tick to remain attached to its animal host—from several hours to several days, depending on the life stage of the tick. It is not difficult to remain on a deer or mouse, for instance, for that amount of time. However, if a tick is attached to a human host, remaining inconspicuous for that amount of time is a challenge.

Like Kyle, the camper who had been bitten by a tick without his knowledge, many people pick up ticks without realizing it. That is because the tick actually injects an anesthetic into the skin as a numbing agent. This makes the bite virtually painless, so unless a person can see the tick at this time, there would be no sharp pain or itching that would indicate the presence of a tick.

In addition to numbing the host's skin, the tick secretes cement-like chemicals in its saliva as it feeds. This cement makes it even more difficult for the tick to come loose from the skin. Finally, the tick's barbed mouth parts inject chemicals that keep the host's blood from clotting and keep the nearby muscles and blood vessels from becoming inflamed. This means that the blood supply continues to flow easily into the tick. Once it has become engorged (ticks consume one hundred times their body weight in blood at a feeding) it drops off the animal—and this, too, is a painless process for the host.

Vectors, Hosts, and Reservoirs

To completely understand Lyme disease, it is important to understand the role played by each part of the chain. Although the deer ticks are what spread the bacteria to people, the Bb bacteria do not originate in the tick. Deer tick larvae are not infected with the Lyme bacteria when they hatch from eggs.

As far as Lyme disease goes, deer ticks are what scientists call vectors. Vectors are simply carriers of a disease who never become sick themselves. The Bb bacteria can live inside the tick, however, and can be passed on by its bite. Ticks become infected with Bb by feeding on the blood of an animal that is already infected with the bacteria—called a reservoir.

In the case of the deer tick, that could be a bird, a rabbit, or a raccoon. However, the most common source of infection is the blood of the white-footed mouse—a rodent that is extremely common in both rural and suburban areas of the Midwest and New England states. When a tick feeds off the blood of the white-footed mouse or one of these other small animals that are infected with Bb and becomes infected itself, it is likely to pass that infection on to other noninfected hosts.

Deer are not reservoirs for Lyme disease. They, like humans, are hosts for the tick. Deer can become infected, but unlike white-footed mice and other reservoirs, their blood cannot infect an uninfected tick. Deer are nonetheless important in the life cycle of the tick, for deer provide the final meal for the adult female ticks before they lay their eggs. Explains one Lyme disease researcher, "Deer are the host of choice for adult ticks. If a female adult tick does not have a blood meal during the summer or fall, it will not be able to produce eggs the next spring. If there are no deer in an area, the number of [deer] ticks will decline over time."[21]

The white-footed mouse is the most common reservoir for Borrelia burgdorferi *bacteria.*

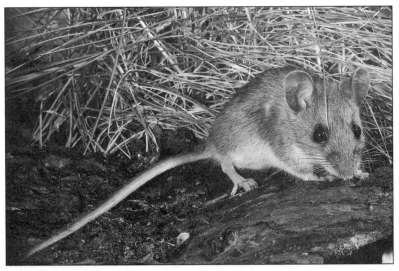

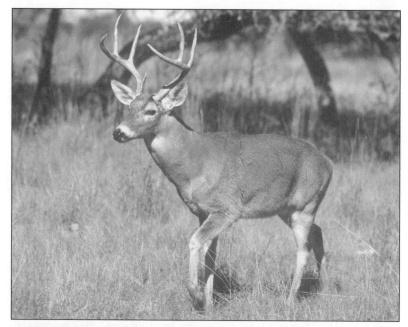

Deer are critical links in the life cycle of a tick. They usually provide the tick its final blood meal before its reproduction stage.

Younger and More Dangerous

Scientists have found that deer ticks are most likely to pass along Lyme disease when they are in the nymph stage. As larvae, they commonly feed on white-footed mice or other small animals during the summer months. If those animals are infected, the blood containing the Bb bacteria passes into the intestinal tracts of the larvae and remains there as the larvae change into nymphs.

The nymphs go all winter without eating, and by the first warm months of spring, they are very active—and hungry. As they go about questing for a blood meal, the Lyme bacteria are still in their intestinal tracts. As a nymph feeds and at the same time releases its chemicals that prevent the blood from coagulating, the bacteria are regurgitated, making their way up through the intestinal tract into the tick's mouth parts. From there, the bacteria pass from the tick to the host. It is at this point where an uninfected animal (including a human) could become infected with Lyme disease. It has been estimated that approximately 80 percent of human Lyme diseases cases are acquired from nymphs.

It is true that the adult ticks may also have residual blood containing Bb in their intestinal tracts. However, scientists maintain that it would be far less likely for a person to become infected by an adult deer tick than from a nymph. For one thing, the time at which the adult tick seeks its final meal is during the cooler weather of middle to late October. Most people are far less likely to be in rural or wooded areas at that time. And those people who are in areas where there are deer ticks would tend to be dressed in clothing that can give some protection from ticks. Finally, because adult ticks are larger than nymphs, they are easier to spot even before they become engorged with blood—in other

While feeding on blood, infected tick nymphs use their barbed mouth parts (pictured) to pass Bb bacteria on to their hosts.

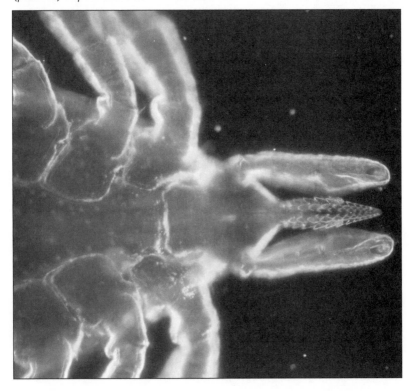

words, these ticks are often detected before the Bb bacteria have a chance to be regurgitated into the host's body.

The Varying Rate of Infection

Not every deer tick is infected with Bb bacteria. In some areas of the United States, between 33 and 48 percent of deer tick nymphs are infected. In other areas, the rate of infected deer ticks is much lower. Obviously, if there is a high percentage of ticks in a particular area, people are more likely to be infected with Lyme disease.

Steve, a resort owner in Wisconsin, knows that he lives in an area where there are many deer ticks. He tries to keep track of the infection rate among ticks for two reasons:

> For one thing, the people who rent out our cabins want to know. And the other reason is that I had Lyme disease once, and I don't want it again. I was lucky—I didn't have it bad. But it's no fun, and it's dangerous if you don't find it early. So we don't take it lightly when we find ticks on us.

> Every so often, the state does a spot check to give people an idea of the rate of infection in their part of the state. It varies, that's for sure. My brother in Minnesota works in an area where the rate is really high—almost 35 percent. Yet twenty miles over, they say that only one in ten ticks is infected. For us last summer, we were told that the rate of infection for our part of the county was about 25 percent. In other words, one out of every four ticks that bites us could have it. Hey—there've been times I come in after mowing and I've got twenty or thirty of the little buggers on me. It's nothing you want to fool with, that's for sure.[22]

Chapter 3

The Signs of Lyme Disease

Just as not every deer tick is infected with the Lyme bacteria, not everyone bitten by an infected tick gets sick. No one is completely sure why; some people's immune systems are evidently able to fight off the infection before they become ill. The vast majority of people bitten by an infected tick do contract Lyme disease, however. And although later symptoms of Lyme disease can vary widely from person to person, there is some consistency in its earliest signs.

The Bull's-Eye Rash

About 70 percent of people who are infected with the Bb bacteria get a strange rash at the site where the tick was attached, appearing anywhere from a few days to a month after the bite. The rash starts as a reddish bump on the skin, much like the bite any tick would leave.

However, as the Bb bacteria push outward from the site, the reddish bump becomes a bigger, dark red circle or oval, caused by increased blood flow to the area. The body is attempting to fight off the increasing numbers of bacteria as they push farther outward from their entry point, multiplying and feeding, seeking new tissue on which to feed.

After several days or weeks, the original red bump often heals, leaving the skin inside the rash lighter in color. This gives the rash a "bull's-eye" look—something seen only with the Lyme bacteria. The rash, which may be warm to the touch and somewhat tender, expands slowly—approximately three-quarters of an inch per day. Some people find that the rash grows only to about two inches in diameter, while on others it can cover an area of skin more than twelve or fourteen inches across.

"It Looked Like the Picture"

Steve, the resort owner, never saw the tick that had attached itself to his chest two years before. However, he did see the reddish bump and watched it carefully.

> I've seen lots of pictures of the rash. We have pamphlets about Lyme disease that show what the rash looks like. So I knew that if that bump—which, by the way, I thought was a spider bite—turned into anything bigger, I had to get in to see the doctor.

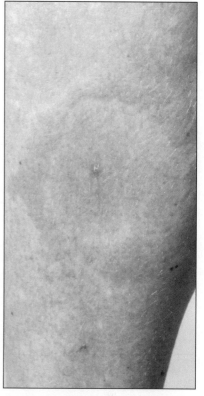

Many people develop a rash where the infected tick was attached. A small, reddish bump usually spreads into a darker ring.

It didn't seem to do anything for almost a week. In fact, I kind of forgot about it after awhile. But then when I was shaving after getting out of the shower, I noticed in the mirror that the bump had definitely turned into a rash. It wasn't real red, but more like what poison ivy looks like, you know? Anyway, it had that light skin inside the rash, and I saw how it looked like the picture—like a bull's eye.

Asked if he felt sick at the time, Steve said no.

> I really didn't feel any different at all. I think that's why it had been so easy to forget about that little bite. It didn't hurt, I didn't

feel sick or tired or any of that. I'll tell you—those pictures helped. You compare your rash to something like that, and you can see if it's similar or not. Because remember, there are all sorts of ticks that bite, that don't give you any disease. I'm not going to run to the doctor over every bite I get.[23]

Not Always Easy to Tell

But for every person such as Steve, whose Lyme disease rash was easy to see, say doctors, there are dozens who never see the bull's-eye rash doctors warn patients about.

Laura, whose son Mike came home from camp with a fever and chills, had no idea that the diagnosis would be Lyme disease.

"He got off the bus saying he was sick," she said. "It was only because he mentioned that he'd had a tick fall out of his hair at camp that I thought we should get him tested. But he didn't have a rash like you see in pictures. They tell you that the sign of Lyme disease is a bull's-eye rash, lighter in the center and red on the outside. But that wasn't Mike."

She explained that Mike has darker pigment to his skin because of his Italian ancestry. "He gets dark, dark brown during the summer. So when I'm looking for a rash, I'm not seeing one. He had something that looked like a bruise on his arm. That was it. I thought, hey, if other people with dark skin decide not to get a Lyme disease test because they don't see that bull's-eye, they could be in trouble."[24]

The Infection Spreads

A person whose only symptom of Lyme disease is the bull's-eye rash is said to be in Stage I of the disease. That means that the infection is local—confined to one area of the body. Doctors agree that Lyme disease is quite easy to cure with antibiotics if it is caught in this first stage. But correctly identifying the rash is often very difficult, if not impossible, to do. The rash is often difficult to see or is misinterpreted as something else. And nearly 20 percent of people with Lyme disease do not get a rash at all. That is why most people with the disease do not even seek medical help while they are in the first stage.

During Stage I, the Bb bacteria in the bloodstream can also cause flulike symptoms, such as fever and chills. Unfortunately, these symptoms, too, are often not serious enough for most people to see a doctor. That, say doctors, is the danger of Lyme disease—and why it is called "the great imitator." Because its symptoms are so similar to those of other illnesses that may go away on their own, there is often no true signal for Lyme disease. Those with the disease, especially in Stage I, are often unaware of the seriousness of their illness. And that gives the disease more time to spread and worsen.

"There are so many times when you can be coming down with some virus, some flu bug or something," said Cherie, the mother of a girl who had Lyme disease. "Most of the time, you just figure you'll get to bed early, take some aspirin and just chill for a day. I don't think I've ever called the doctor unless things have gotten worse. I mean, if everybody that felt under the weather like that demanded doctor appointments, there wouldn't be time for the clinics to see anyone else, right?"

Cherie's daughter had not had a rash, and the first of the symptoms of Lyme disease were fever and body aches. Cherie, who had been a nurse for seven years, was convinced it was something minor.

"She'd been sneezing a bit just before she became feverish," said Cherie.

And so we thought the fever was just part of that. So we watched it for a week. After that time, she wasn't showing any sign of getting over it, so I took her in. The doctor said they'd seen a lot of flu, and thought it was just a stubborn case. A week later, no improvement, and we saw another doctor, and he gave her two tests—one for strep and one for mono. But both were negative. After a while, we weren't sure what to think.[25]

Stage II

If untreated during Stage I of the disease, the Bb bacteria continue to spread through the body. The bacteria may attack a particular organ, one of the body's systems, or joints, such as knees or elbows. Doctors refer to this as Stage II of Lyme disease—a

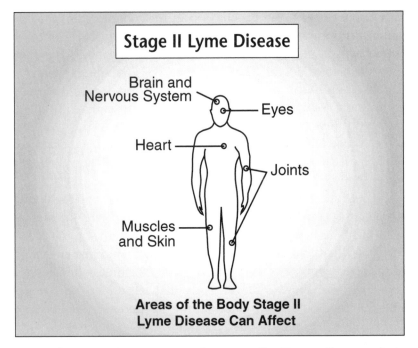

Stage II Lyme Disease

Brain and
Nervous System

Eyes

Heart

Joints

Muscles
and Skin

**Areas of the Body Stage II
Lyme Disease Can Affect**

time when problems worsen dramatically. Depending on their individual body chemistry and metabolism, some patients remain in Stage I for several weeks or longer, while others can proceed to Stage II symptoms within several days. However, why the bacteria spread to the knees of one patient and to an organ in another during Stage II remains a mystery to researchers.

During this second stage, between 10 and 20 percent of Lyme disease patients experience heart problems. This might mean irregular heartbeats or chest pain. Sometimes heart problems are triggered by the rapid increase in white blood cells, which the body produces in response to any infection. As one doctor explains, the presence of so many cells can cause swelling in the heart muscle itself: "The white blood cells increase in numbers, and the spaces between cells swell with fluid. This inflammation of the heart's muscles can reduce the strength of the heart's contractions, and in this condition the heart cannot sustain the same load it normally would."[26]

When this happens, the person becomes fatigued much more easily and experiences shortness of breath or dizzy spells. And while doctors are always concerned when there are problems with the heart, the condition when associated with Lyme disease is almost never fatal. In fact, fewer than ten Lyme patients have died from heart infections as of October 2001. Once antibiotics take effect, the heart's rhythm and strength usually return to normal.

Bell's Palsy

If the Bb bacteria get into the nervous system by attacking the spinal cord or the brain, a person may develop Bell's palsy, which is a weakening of the facial muscles. In most cases, just one side of the face is affected: The right side of the mouth can smile while the left side is almost paralyzed, for example.

Joe, whose Stage II symptoms came on less than two weeks after he was bitten by a deer tick, said that Bell's palsy was one of the strangest of the symptoms he experienced. "I lost control of the nerves on the left side of my face," he said. "My eye drooped, and my lip, too. I couldn't eat right—I couldn't swallow easily. Really, I ate like a caveman—food would get caught in my gums, it was awful. Bell's palsy doesn't last, but it feels so odd."[27]

Some patients with Bell's palsy find that only one eye can make tears, and that they can only hear out of one ear. Many have trouble talking because the nerves to the tongue are affected by the bacteria. "Some people say they feel like they've had a stroke," said one medical worker. "They have trouble making certain speech sounds—especially 'th' or 'sh'. And they get embarrassed because they know they don't sound right, or even look the way they always did."[28]

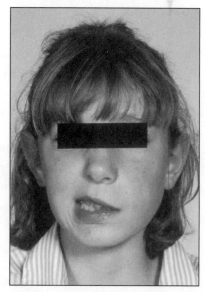

Bell's palsy, a weakening of the facial muscles, is a Stage II symptom that can occur if Bb bacteria attack the nervous system.

"I Couldn't Make Myself Go to the Meeting"

There are other symptoms of infection in the nervous system, too. Rich knew there was something wrong when he began having severe back pains, which radiated down both of his legs. Although he had a history of back pain, this was unlike anything he'd experienced before.

> None of the usual things worked. Hot packs, aspirin, baths, changing position frequently. It did nothing at all. I tried to work through it, you know, but that came to an end when I was in New York for some meetings. I sat up in bed on Friday in the hotel, and I hurt so badly I was almost crying. I couldn't make myself go to the meeting, I was just in too much pain. I got a plane back home and went straight to the doctor's office. I asked him to do a Lyme test, partly because a friend of mine had just been diagnosed with it. And the test was positive.[29]

Invading the Brain

When the Lyme bacteria invade the brain itself, a number of other symptoms can occur—some of them very frightening. As the white blood cells rush to the brain to aid in fighting the infection, there is swelling around various blood vessels. This can interfere with the normal passage of blood. Without a steady supply of blood, the nerve cells are unable to function, and a patient's ability to think and reason may be affected.

Joe noticed that he was having trouble concentrating when he had Lyme disease. "I'm a business lawyer," he explained. "And I write a lot of contracts, things like that—so inability to concentrate is definitely a problem. But I really was finding it hard to stay focused. I was losing my train of thought in the middle of something. I had trouble remembering things I normally would never forget. I even had trouble with the physical act of writing."[30]

Hilary, whose father struggled for years with Lyme disease, said that his brain was affected so dramatically that his entire personality changed. An intelligent, gregarious man before catching Lyme disease, he quickly became disoriented, depressed, and agitated.

He would not keep his clothes on, and his speech became difficult to understand. He was so disruptive [in the hospital] to the other patients that he was moved to the psych unit. There he was straightjacketed and given drugs to "calm him down." . . . [Eventually] he lost the ability to swallow food, recognize family members, and speak. His behavior was violent, yet he was completely unaware of his surroundings.[31]

Lyme Arthritis

In addition to heart and nervous system disorders, Stage II Lyme disease can result in severe swelling and pain in the joints and tendons, which are the tissues that connect bones. This condition is often called Lyme arthritis—pain that can make it difficult to do even the simplest things.

Ronald, a forty-three-year-old driving instructor, found the arthritis and the fatigue that accompanied it the worst part of Lyme disease. He said, "Your will to do anything—shave, tie your shoelaces—just dissolves. . . . It is grinding, debilitating, and absolutely devastating."[32]

In many Stage II cases, Lyme arthritis attacks the victim's knees, resulting in severe swelling and pain in the joints and tendons.

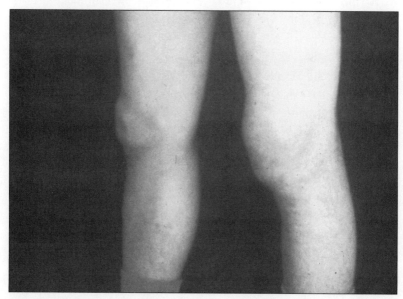

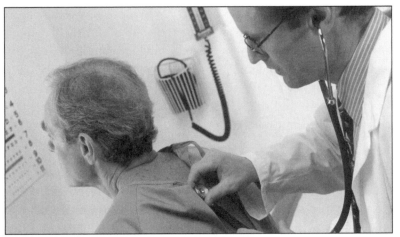

Known as "the great imitator," Lyme disease has a long history of baffling the medical community and of being misdiagnosed.

For reasons yet unknown, children with Stage II Lyme disease are most apt to experience Lyme arthritis. And in more than 90 percent of these cases, it is the knees that are affected. In her book, Polly Murray documents the problem that occurred with two of her sons when they became infected with Lyme disease:

> Wednesday, March 24—Gil's left knee was swollen, his left elbow hurt, and the left side of his neck was tender. He had to resort to using crutches. . . . Todd was still on crutches and having headaches as well. His shoulder hurt, and the knee swelling was the same. . . . Monday March 29—Todd's shoulder hurt and his knee was the same. Gil was still on crutches and he was keeping his knee elevated as much as he could. The swelling had advanced into his thigh, and his left calf also hurt. His left ankle was so swollen that you couldn't see the ankle bone.[33]

By the time victims of Lyme disease are in Stage II, the symptoms are painful and often even frightening, and the victims almost always seek medical help. Unfortunately, many patients find that the medical community has had a great deal of difficulty diagnosing Lyme disease, and the relief and reassurance patients seek from their doctors do not always come as quickly as they had hoped.

Chapter 4

Diagnosis and Treatment

Positively diagnosing Lyme disease—especially in Stage I—is very tricky, for several reasons. For one thing, the early symptoms—tick bite and bull's-eye rash—are not found in every case. In addition, more than half of sufferers cannot recall being bitten by a tick.

Horses, Not Zebras

In his book, *Lyme Disease: The Cause, the Cure, the Controversy*, Dr. Alan Barbour explains that doctors are trained to find the most probable explanation for any patient's illness, based on a symptom. Says Barbour, "One of the enduring aphorisms of medicine (in North America, at least), is this: If you hear hoofbeats outside the house, think of horses, not zebras."[34]

For a doctor evaluating a patient with body aches and fever, who cannot remember a tick bite or who does not have a bull's-eye rash, a diagnosis of Lyme disease is the least probable cause—a zebra. There are simply too many more common explanations for the patient's symptoms, say doctors.

However, there are many patients who complain that their doctors were reluctant to even consider Lyme disease as an explanation for their illness. One woman told her doctor she had pulled a tick from her skin and asked whether her constant muscle aches and fever could be signs of Lyme disease. She was told no, that she had a virus. Even after several months without relief from the symptoms, and despite repeated requests to do further tests for Lyme disease, the doctor did not think it was necessary to consider that possibility.

43

A man who had had high fevers, a swollen eye, and sharp pains in his abdomen and temple suspected Lyme disease, too. When he noticed a rash while in the bathtub, he says he was almost relieved, for it was an explanation for his problems. "[The rash] was on the back of my left leg, and it was bright, bright red," he said. "I thought, okay, this is Lyme. I've got the rash and now they can diagnose what I've got. So I go in the next day and show the doctor, and he isn't convinced. He says it's not the bull's eye."[35]

Proof from the Lab?

Because there is so much ambiguity in Lyme disease symptoms, doctors hoped that a blood test could tell with certainty whether a patient had the disease. For many illnesses, a simple blood test can determine the nature of a problem. "That's the thing about Lyme disease," said the mother of one Lyme patient.

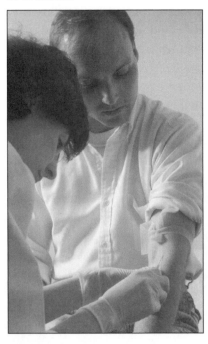

Drawing a patient's blood (pictured) is sometimes the first step in identifying Lyme disease bacteria, but recognizing Bb is difficult.

It's not clear-cut, like some things are. We get spoiled by what doctors and technicians can do on an everyday basis. I can take my son in because he has a sore throat. The doctor . . . sends the lab tech in and she can take a swab of the junk at the back of his throat and take it back to the lab. In a few minutes they can tell if he's got strep throat. Just like that—it's easy, like connect-the-dots. But it's not like that with Lyme.[36]

There are tests that can be done, but their results can sometimes be inaccurate. Yet without an alternative, many doctors utilize the most common method of laboratory test-

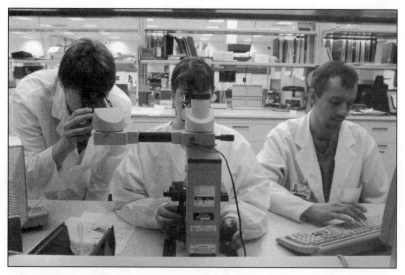

Laboratory technicians test blood samples for Borrelia burgdorferi *bacteria.*

ing—the blood test. However, the blood tests for finding evidence of Lyme disease are very different from blood tests for other illnesses.

Antibodies

The main reason that laboratory tests for Lyme disease are not always accurate is that the Bb bacterium that causes the disease is very difficult to isolate. Doctors cannot view the bacterium from a patient's blood or tissue sample as they can the bacterium that causes strep throat, for example. The nature of Bb, writes one researcher, is that it is "infamous for its ability to transform its appearance chemically, in much the same way a criminal might change clothes and hair color to avoid detection and capture."[37]

Since it is almost impossible to measure the number of Bb bacteria in a patient's blood, laboratory tests instead target antibodies in the blood. Anytime infection is present in the body, the immune system produces special proteins, called antibodies, whose job is to locate and attach themselves to the infecting bacteria or viruses. After attaching themselves to the intruders, the antibodies help the body's white blood cells to eliminate them.

Each group of antibodies is different; those produced to fight a cold differ in chemical makeup from those antibodies produced to fight measles or chicken pox. If a test of a patient's blood found evidence of Lyme disease antibodies, then it would mean that that patient had Lyme disease. However, the answers provided by the antibodies test are not so clear-cut.

Difficulties with Blood Tests

The antibodies test is relatively simple to administer. A sample of blood is drawn from a patient into a glass tube. The tube is put on a machine that spins it around quickly, a process that separates the dark red blood cells from the light-yellow-colored fluid in the blood called serum. It is the serum that contains antibodies, and when a certain chemical dye is added to the serum, Lyme disease antibodies can be seen.

There are definite drawbacks to the antibodies tests currently available. The most important drawback is that the tests are often inaccurate. Sometimes the results give a false positive—indicating

A chemical dye is applied to test tubes of blood serum to uncover Lyme disease antibodies. This process, unfortunately, is often inaccurate.

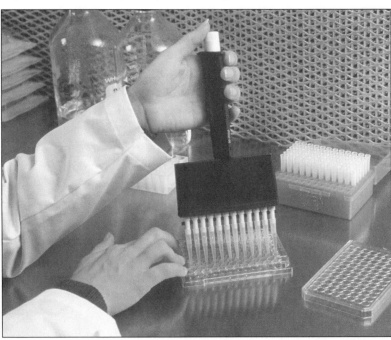

the presence of Lyme antibodies when the patient does not have the disease. This sometimes occurs when a person still has antibodies from a previous infection—and the test is unable to tell the difference between those antibodies and Lyme disease antibodies.

More common are false negatives—results that show no evidence of Lyme antibodies, even though the patient really has the disease. There are several reasons for false negative results, but the most likely is that the patient's body has not manufactured enough antibodies to show up on the test. After someone is bitten by an infected deer tick, it usually takes several weeks before the body begins producing the antibodies; in fact, even when the bull's-eye rash appears, it is rare for a test to detect antibodies.

Comparing Test Results

Most Lyme specialists agree that an antibodies test has the best chance of picking up the Bb antibodies from six to eight weeks after the tick bite. Unfortunately, by that time the infection has spread into other parts of the body, becoming Stage II Lyme disease—which is far more difficult to cure.

"That's so ironic," said one man who has had Lyme disease,

> because the whole idea of getting a blood test is to catch [the disease] early, so you can treat it and cure it. And you go in, and a lot of times even though you are sure you got bit by a deer tick and you feel like there's a good chance you've got it, and then your test comes back negative. And the doctor says, "Hey, I got no evidence you've got Lyme disease, and I can't write you a prescription for an antibiotic that you don't need." Then he says, "Come back in four weeks and maybe the test will show something." But by then, the disease will have spread and it won't be easy to cure. It makes no sense![38]

Many doctors agree. Because of the false readings of antibodies tests, they have begun changing the way they look at the tests. Instead of using it as a final proof that someone with Lyme disease symptoms actually has the disease, they administer the test as one more piece of evidence. Doctors who suspect Lyme disease might order the test just to confirm what they already suspect. Experts say that a doctor needs to be aware that the tests are not foolproof. Doctors must rely on the patient's symptoms—as well as the likelihood of Lyme disease exposure—in addition to the blood test before making a diagnosis.

Other Testing

Sometimes a diagnosis of Lyme disease is mostly a matter of eliminating other possibilities. Rich, who cut short his business trip to New York because of severe pains in his back and legs, was given a blood antibodies test for Lyme disease, which came up positive. A neurologist (a doctor who specializes in diseases of the nervous system) explained to Rich that the Lyme test sometimes results in false positives.

> He wanted to make absolutely sure that my pain wasn't being caused by anything structural, you know? Maybe a pinched nerve, or a slipped disc or even a tumor, I guess—something like that. Any of those things could have been responsible for my symptoms. And rather than put me on medication which wouldn't

The antibodies test is sometimes followed up by a spinal tap (pictured) in which doctors take fluid from around the spinal cord and examine it for Bb.

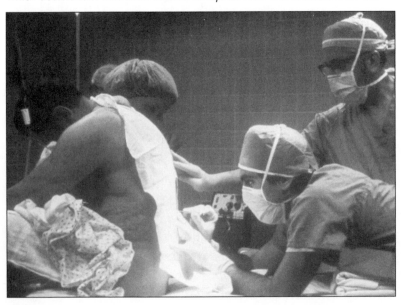

help if I didn't have Lyme disease, they wanted to make sure. And so I had an MRI [magnetic resonance imaging] where they insert you into a big tube, and scan you for all those problems.

Rich said the experience was terrible.

Not only was I in a lot of pain, but I'm also claustrophobic. And after four hours of MRI, I had had more than enough. The good news, though, is that they ruled out anything structural. What they did see, though, were that all my nerve endings there by my spinal cord were inflamed, so that was another hint that I had an infection.

In Rich's case, doctors were able to do a more specific test for Lyme disease since it was in his nervous system. "They did a spinal tap," he explained, "where they take fluid from around your spine and examine it for signs of Lyme disease. And they found signs of Lyme bacteria, which confirmed the first test as being accurate."[39]

Medications for Lyme Disease

Doctors are not sure why, but some people infected with Lyme disease produce antibodies in their bodies which can fight off the infection without medication. Most cases, however, will not go away without treatment, and once it is determined that a patient has Lyme disease, the doctor will prescribe some form of antibiotic. Doctors treating Lyme disease orally choose either amoxicillin, which is a type of penicillin, or a tetracycline drug, such as doxycycline. If one is not effective, or if a patient experiences a side effect, like an upset stomach, a doctor can switch to the other.

There are various choices of antibiotics, and they differ slightly from one another. Some are best for Stage I, when the disease is more localized. Others are best for Stage II, because they can penetrate various tissues of the body where the bacteria may be hiding. Some medications are best for children, while others are best for women who are pregnant. Tetracycline drugs, for example, can cause permanent discoloration of a child's teeth, so a doctor might avoid prescribing them for a child.

Each type of antibiotic works in its own way. For example, antibiotics of the penicillin family kill the bacteria outright. The Bb bacterium needs to build a sturdy, protective wall around itself to survive, and penicillin destroys the wall. "When the cell walls of the bacteria are weakened," explains one doctor, "the bacteria literally burst at the seams. The numbers of bacteria can drop a hundredfold, a thousandfold, or even a millionfold within the first day of treatment."[40] Antibiotics from the tetracycline family, on the other hand, do not kill the bacteria directly. Instead, they prevent them from growing or forming DNA that enables the bacteria to reproduce.

Antibiotics work together with the body's own disease-fighting system. By holding down the growth of the invading bacteria, the antibiotic can give the body time to produce the large numbers of antibodies needed to fight the infection.

Sometimes Pills Are Not Enough

A patient with Stage I Lyme disease usually can be cured with three to four weeks' worth of antibiotics, usually in pill form. However, if the disease has begun to spread to other parts of the body, the

Large doses of antibiotics are administered intravenously to a Lyme disease patient.

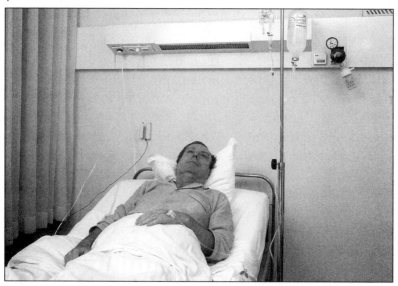

cure will almost always take more time. Many patients with Stage II Lyme disease stay on the medication for at least four to six weeks.

In certain cases, when the Lyme bacteria have invaded the heart or the nervous system, it is important to get the medication into the bloodstream quickly, and in very strong doses. Pills that strong would lose some of their strength as they are digested in the body, and the strong ingredients would almost certainly result in an upset stomach or other digestive ailment. For that reason, doctors sometimes hospitalize a patient and order that the drugs be given intravenously: Medicine in liquid form is dripped slowly from a tube to a hollow needle that has been inserted in the patient's vein.

The Hospital and Beyond

Intravenous (IV) medication is almost always begun in a hospital. That way, doctors and nurses can be sure that the patient is responding to the medication and that the amount of each dose is correct. "That's what happened to me," said Rich. "They put me in the hospital right away after they found the [Lyme] bacteria from the spinal tap. They explained that when it's in the nervous system, it's really hard to contain with oral antibiotics, so I was put on IVs for thirty days."

Rich said that it was three or four days until he noticed improvement in the severe back and leg pain he had with the disease. By then, the doctors allowed him to go home. "I'm still doing the IVs—even out of the hospital," he said, rolling up his shirtsleeve to reveal an IV tube and needle taped securely to the skin on his arm.

"This is the greatest thing—a delivery system for the medicine that stays in my arm here for the whole time I'm on IVs. When it's time for me to get my dose, I insert the medicine in here," he says, pointing to the tube. "This way, the medicine goes right into the vein into my heart where it's pumped through my body. It doesn't hurt—I do feel the medicine after I inject it, because it's kept in the refrigerator and it gets pretty cold. But there's no pain."

He smiled. "And really, it's been great, because it allows me to be home with my family getting well, instead of lying in a hospital bed. And after the thirty days are up, the doctor will remove this setup, and hopefully, I'll be all done."[41]

Chapter 5

The Most Serious Lyme Disease

In many cases, Lyme disease is cured quickly—the patient finishes the prescribed medication and the symptoms disappear. However, there are some people who do not get better. Their symptoms, which may lessen while being treated with medication, inevitably return in a stronger, more debilitating form called chronic Lyme disease. If Stage I and Stage II are untreated, Lyme disease may progress to this third stage. For some people, the disease has even proved fatal. For a great many others, it has made life for them and their families a nightmare—physically, financially, and emotionally.

Life-Threatening

While Stage I and Stage II are almost never life-threatening, chronic Lyme may be. Sometimes a case becomes life-threatening by the nature of the area of the body attacked by the Bb bacteria—someone that has the Lyme disease bacteria settle in the heart or the brain, for example. The danger is sometimes compounded if the patient has another serious medical condition. A person with diabetes, who already has trouble with constricted or blocked blood vessels, may be in real danger of suffering a stroke or heart attack if Lyme bacteria invade the cardiovascular system.

The dangers have been compounded because of the limitations of medical knowledge about the disease—especially when it was first identified. It was not immediately understood, for example, that Lyme disease could be transmitted from a pregnant woman to her unborn child.

Jamie Forschner was six years old when he died from chronic Lyme disease. He had been infected before he was born, when his mother Karen was bitten by a tick. When Karen asked her doctor whether her infection posed any danger to her unborn child, she was told that he could not become infected while in the womb. However, as Karen now says, "Jamie died from a disease the nation's medical and scientific communities thought he could not get. They were wrong."

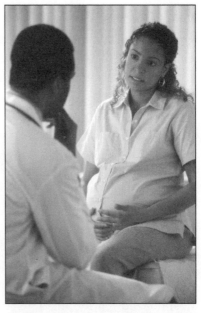

Doctors have only recently discovered that pregnant mothers are capable of transmitting Lyme disease to their unborn children.

Too Late

Karen and her husband knew, when their infant son was only six weeks old, that he had severe health problems. "[H]e had begun to vomit repeatedly," she wrote, "and had alarming eye tremors, a sign of brain infection."[42] As the months went by, Jamie developed heart problems, blindness, and deafness. He suffered from Bell's palsy and signs of brain damage.

When tests showed that Jamie had Lyme bacteria in his system, he was put on antibiotics. However, because the disease had spread throughout his system, the medicine could provide only temporary relief from some of his symptoms. Frustrated, Karen felt certain that had they known that Lyme disease could be passed from mother to unborn child, they might have identified his problems far earlier. "If Jamie had been treated right away," she said in 1989, "he might not be the mess he has become."[43]

However, the little boy could not overcome the disease that ravaged his body. With the infection causing swelling and inflammation in his brain, Jamie experienced seizures and died in June 1991.

An Ongoing Infection

Fortunately, fatalities from Lyme disease have been rare. But chronic Lyme disease—which is the ongoing presence of symptoms sometimes even after treatment—occurs with frightening frequency. Just as Lyme disease can become life-threatening in some cases, it can progress to a chronic stage if it is not treated early. It is estimated that between 10 and 15 percent of people with Lyme disease will be in that category—still showing symptoms after they finish their treatment.

Chronic Lyme disease is marked most often by constant fatigue that does not diminish even with sleep. Headaches—especially those brought on by bright light—and ongoing arthritis are very common symptoms, too. Many people find that their muscles cramp severely and that they lose muscle tone. One Canadian woman had been treated with medications but was hospitalized ten months later when pains in her legs and other symptoms of arthritis made it impossible for her to walk without a cane. "I was a healthy person," she said, "and all of a sudden, I couldn't get out of bed or even walk."[44]

For some sufferers of chronic Lyme disease, the hardest part has been learning to think of their condition as almost a way of life, rather than a passing infection. "It's the way I live now," said one man. "Sometimes I can't even remember what a day without headaches and swollen joints feels like."[45]

Children at Risk

Though any person can develop a case of chronic Lyme disease, researchers have found that children in general are especially at risk for chronic Lyme disease. More than 50 percent of Lyme infections involve children under the age of twelve; of those, the largest percentage of children suffering from Lyme disease are under the age of five.

It is distressingly common, say pediatricians, to find that many of these young Lyme patients are in the chronic stage by the time they are diagnosed. The reason for this may be that young children are not able to verbalize their symptoms, as

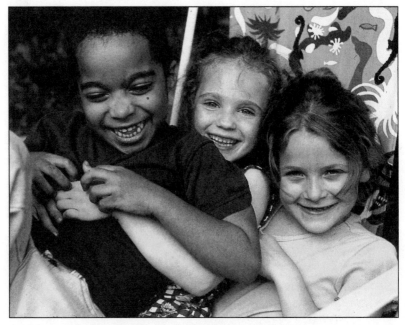

Children under the age of twelve have the highest risk of developing chronic Lyme disease.

adults are. What may indeed be the flulike symptoms of Stage I Lyme or muscle and joint pains may be misunderstood by parents as tiredness, teething, colic, or the onset of a cold.

Experts say that sometimes children who do complain of chronic pain are frequently scolded for complaining or inventing their symptoms. However, says pediatric Lyme disease specialist Dr. Louis Corsaro, parents and teachers should be aware that children are very truthful about whether they feel sick:

> Children don't lie when it comes to aches and pains, and they don't exaggerate. It should be easy to tell when a child is really ill because they only have two speeds—sleep and fast. As a pediatrician in an area where I've handled more than 1,200 cases of Lyme—350 of those in the chronic stage—there is no question in my mind that if a diagnosis is made early, short-term antibiotics are effective. But if children are dismissed as complainers . . . the child can go into a chronic stage, which is much more difficult to treat.[46]

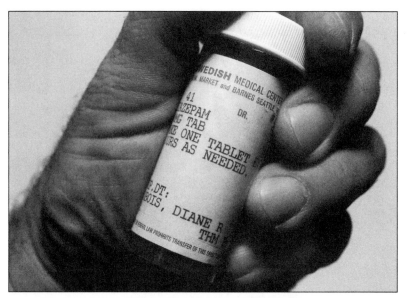

Prescribing the correct dosage of an antibiotic is often difficult and must be considered on a case-by-case basis.

Not Long Enough on Medication

Some experts feel that many cases of chronic Lyme disease—in children as well as in adults—result from too short a regimen of medication. Normally, when a patient with Stage I or early Stage II Lyme disease is diagnosed, a physician prescribes three to four weeks of antibiotic treatment. However, there are many cases in which the patient is still experiencing symptoms after that time.

Kathleen, who was diagnosed with Lyme disease in May 2000, was considerably better after her three weeks on medication. "I had the flu symptoms," she explained,

> and the rash—although mine wasn't the classic bull's-eye that the literature talks about. Anyway, my doctor put me on an antibiotic for 21 days, and I really started feeling better pretty quickly.
>
> I had been achy and running a fever in the afternoons, and had been having headaches. But all that stopped by about the fifth day on my medication. I was really careful to keep taking it, though—my doctor made a big deal out of the fact that too

many people stop taking medicine after they feel better. She said I needed to finish the whole bottle, the whole three weeks. So I did."

Lyme Returns—and Worse

Kathleen said that she felt pretty well after the three weeks on medication, although she was still fairly tired. "I wasn't sick," she insisted.

> I just felt my limits, I guess you could say. Where before Lyme disease I could work out at the gym before going to work and feel energized, if I went to the gym, I felt like I could maybe go home and take a nap. I got tired quicker.

> But after a couple of weeks, I started going downhill. My achiness came back, and although I wasn't running a fever, I had a lot of headaches. Noises seemed to bother me more than usual—it was like all of a sudden, my hearing was way too sensitive. I went back to my doctor, thinking maybe she'd put me on more medicine, or a stronger one or something. But she wouldn't. She told me that what I was having were temporary symptoms, and that more medication wouldn't help that at all.

After two more weeks of symptoms that continued to get worse, Kathleen went to a different doctor. She said,

> I didn't get the feeling my doctor understood how bad I really felt. So this new doctor put me on a different antibiotic, and after four weeks, I felt better. I kind of waited to see if I'd relapse like before, but I was okay. I really wish [my first doctor] had listened to me—I had to go through weeks of feeling lousy for nothing.[47]

Each Case Is Different

Experts are not yet certain why some cases of Lyme disease do not respond to the normal length of antibiotic treatment. Some believe that the disease may have begun to spread in the body, doing more damage than at first understood. In cases such as

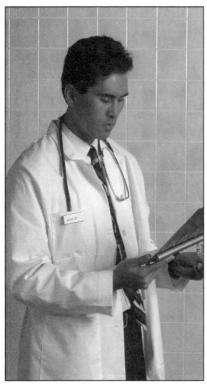

Carefully studying each patient's medical chart may prove crucial when deciding how to treat a particular case of Lyme disease.

these, doctors may have thought they were treating Stage I disease, when in fact they were faced with a Stage II infection, which would require more aggressive treatment, such as intravenous medications administered in the hospital.

Other doctors maintain that even with such aggressive treatment, some cases just are more difficult to treat—and research has been done that supports that view. Dr. Paul Lavoie, a Lyme disease researcher, explained that the bacteria can survive for a long time in some patients, even though those patients may feel initially that they are getting better:

I have found evidence for persistent infection in improved patients with ongoing antibiotic therapy of a few years. This supports the concept that a bacteriologic cure is not easily achieved by current therapies and that we must not dismiss our patients' complaints following even very prolonged therapy. We must keep an open mind.[48]

Problems with Chronic Lyme Disease

As more studies have been done on the effects of chronic Lyme disease, doctors are beginning to see that patients often experience new symptoms, too—not just a worsening of the original symptoms of the disease. Many of these new symptoms, say experts, are caused by the bacteria's effects on the brain. Memory loss, an inability to concentrate, and confusion—sometimes referred to as "Lyme fog"—are often ongoing problems for a chronic sufferer.

Lisa, twenty-three, was only a semester away from getting her Ph.D. in psychology when she became sick with Lyme disease. Unfortunately, by the time doctors were able to identify the cause of her symptoms, the disease had progressed to the chronic stage. As she explained, Lyme fog and the frustration that accompanies it have made her life very difficult:

> I feel like everything is surreal and that I am not actually here. . . . It feels as if [I] cannot concentrate and that I am about two seconds behind everyone. But nothing helps. I feel like I am trapped in my head when I get that foggy feeling. . . . I feel as if I am going to pass out, dizziness in my brain, which makes me perspire and feel as if I'm going to black out, ringing in my ears which sounds more like a whooshing sound.[49]

"It Feels Like a Galaxy Away"

As the years of treatment add up, feelings of isolation and hopelessness can accompany chronic Lyme disease for many young adults.

But one of the worst aspects of the disease is the feeling of hopelessness and isolation many chronic Lyme disease patients experience. Cynthia, an eighteen-year-old from Kentucky, has dealt with those feelings for eight years. IV treatments that lasted for months at a time made school attendance spotty, she recalled. "The kids I went to school with didn't know anything about my problems; therefore, they didn't want to have much to do with me. That really hurt me, more than the disease did."[50]

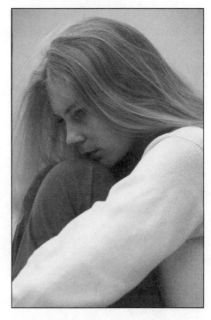

But the feelings of isolation affect adults, too. "A lot of it is having to deal with a disease not too many people understand—including doctors," said David. "You spend so much time going to different specialists or clinics, telling your symptoms to different people, you start burning out. I know I just got to the point of feeling like I was on my own. Nobody except me understands how I feel. Maybe twenty years from now, people will have an easy time getting diagnosed, getting treated. Now it's hell."[51]

Rafelle, whose Lyme disease was not diagnosed for twelve years, agreed. Suffering from depression and guilt because she felt like a burden to her family, she said that her problems were almost too numerous to count. She felt sad because it was not long before that she had had a much different view of herself. "I was an energetic, funny, and lighthearted person," she said. "It's a challenge to preserve some of these traits, and impossible for others. . . . It feels like a galaxy away, that I would ever feel like the true me again."[52]

Chapter 6

Beyond the Symptoms

In addition to its painful and debilitating symptoms, Lyme disease has caused a number of other serious problems for those who suffer from it—especially those whose Lyme disease is ongoing. For many of these patients, the enormous emotional and financial burdens of the disease have become overwhelming.

A Long Process of Diagnosis

Lyme disease patients insist that it is not always the treatment itself that is costly. One 1993 study, conducted by the Lyme Disease Foundation, looked into the costs of Lyme disease, and the results were staggering. The study examined the cases of five hundred patients who had been diagnosed by a physician and found that on average, each patient had had to see five doctors (including various specialists) before getting a correct diagnosis. In addition, the study determined that the average total of a patient's medical bills before being diagnosed was $14,797.

These facts would not surprise Liz, a nurse and the mother of a teenager who was diagnosed with Lyme disease. She said that her daughter saw twice that many doctors, and the expense was enormous:

> I scanned my checkbook (can't have a test without a check!) and was able to add up an interesting history before Katie was diagnosed. She saw ten M.D.'s (that we recall) and had three upper endoscopies, one colonoscopy, one lumbar puncture, three upper GI [gastrointestinal] series, one ultrasound, one

CAT scan, one MRI, two small bowel series, and blood work done over thirty times.[53]

After Diagnosis

The bills can quickly mount after patients are diagnosed. If they are lucky, a Lyme disease test, a few weeks' worth of medication, and a follow-up visit to the doctor will be the extent of their cost—approximately $250. However, for those whose illness is in Stage II or does not disappear after the antibiotic treatment, or for those who suffer a relapse in the weeks after the treatment, the costs are extremely high. Those whose cases required hospitalization and long regimens of IV antibiotics had costs that were $100,000 or more.

Marie Ciasullo and three of her children of Fairfield County, Connecticut, have suffered from chronic Lyme disease for more than seven years. The costs, which so far have run into the hundreds of thousands of dollars, have been overwhelming to Marie

For some Lyme disease sufferers, paying medical bills accrued during treatment is a serious financial strain.

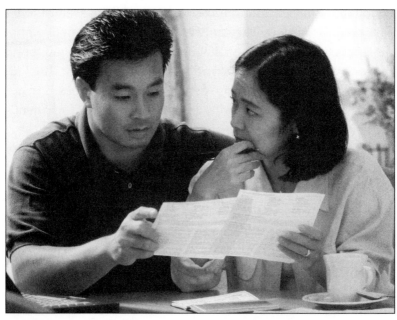

and her husband—the only one in the family who has avoided the disease. She said openly, "He and I live on the edge of financial disaster, due to Lyme disease."[54]

One man said that his bills were so high that he was unable to keep up his house payments. "It was really stressful," he said. "Every month, the doctor bills, the specialists, the tests—all that stuff that was so expensive—it would come rolling in. I would be lying inside, feeling sick, and I'd hear the mailman come, you know—that little clink of the mail slot? And I remember I'd get this clenching feeling in my chest, like I knew it was more bills that I couldn't pay."[55]

Hanging Onto a Job

The financial strain is much more severe because so many patients are forced to cut back on work. The 1993 study estimated that before being diagnosed, the average lost income for a Lyme disease patient was $7,877. After diagnosis, the lost income averaged about $6,500. However, the lost income from work is far higher in Stage II or chronic Lyme disease.

Many people find that the disease makes it impossible for them to continue with their jobs. David, who had worked for six years as a landscaper, was unable to keep up with the physical demands of his job. "I couldn't lift a shovel after awhile," he said. "And even driving the truck to the job site was hard, turning the steering wheel was painful for my shoulders. I tried to keep working as long as I could—if nothing else, than for the health benefits. But it was too much for me."[56]

The inability to work is not only a physical problem—some patients with Lyme whose nervous systems are affected can no longer work because of the loss of memory or cognitive skills. A teacher who can no longer remember how to explain a simple math problem, a doctor who cannot recall how to explain a procedure to a patient, a secretary who can no longer spell or operate her computer—these are all patients who cannot work. Mary, a head nurse in a busy psychiatric ward, recalled how her performance slipped noticeably. "My documentation [of patients] began to seem nonsensical, and I had to reread everything I had

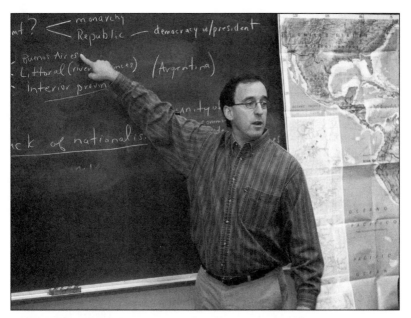

Maintaining steady work habits and on-the-job focus is difficult for many Lyme disease patients.

written and correct it. . . . I had difficulty finding the right word, and often forgot what I was going to say mid-sentence."[57]

For many, the effects of Lyme almost resembled Alzheimer's disease. "My wife," said one New York man, "used to be a tenured professor of mathematics at SUNY [State University of New York]. Now she can't leave the house because she won't be able to find her way back."[58]

Tim, a New Jersey lumberyard manager, recalled being frightened by the rapid mental changes he was seeing in himself because of Lyme disease: "I would forget to do simple things at work; make mistakes that a new worker would make but not a manager—like wrong count on supplies, and lumber—the wrong length. I would invert numbers, left for right. . . . My boss told me to resign as manager or be fired."[59]

"I Couldn't Give My Boss an Honest Answer"

Sometimes employers are willing to be patient and wait for the employee to feel better or for necessary skills to return. However, for many, the on-again, off-again nature of ongoing Lyme disease means that there are no guarantees when a patient will feel well enough to return to work.

"I couldn't give my boss an honest answer," said one woman. "Every Friday I'd call and I'd just say, 'I hope I'll be in Monday.' But then Monday would come and I'd have some new symptom, or an old one would come back. Finally, [my boss] just said, 'I gotta find someone else.' I know he felt bad, and I understood. But at the same time, I'm thinking, 'How in the world am I going to survive?'"[60]

The loss of a job is a critical problem not only because it is a loss of income. In many cases, the health benefits provided by an employer are the only way patients can afford medical care. Once those benefits are gone, many Lyme disease sufferers are forced to stop their treatment, since paying out of pocket for such expensive procedures is almost always beyond people's budgets. However, the decision to stop treatment can sometimes have grave consequences.

Chronic Lyme disease brings with it a great deal of uncertainty for patients dealing with long-term treatments.

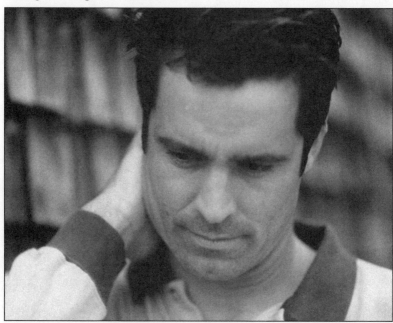

Dangerous Decisions

In her book, *Coping with Lyme Disease: A Practical Guide to Dealing with Diagnosis and Treatment,* Denise Lang tells about Kevin, a Lyme sufferer whose wife and twelve-year-old daughter also had the disease. When his insurance company discontinued their coverage of the family, the family suspended treatment, hoping that their time on antibiotics had eliminated the Bb bacteria from their bodies. However, writes Lang, "All three family members began sliding backward when treatment was stopped. . . . [Kevin's] daughter began having tremors and heart palpitations, which landed her in the hospital."

Because they could not both continue their own treatment while paying the high costs of their daughter's hospitalization, Kevin and his wife discontinued their medication. Ironically, however, while the daughter's health greatly improved, both Kevin and his wife suffered setbacks. Writes Lang, "Today Kevin . . . is in a wheelchair; his wife uses a cane. Their daughter is off IV therapy and on

In extreme cases of chronic Lyme disease, failing to take antibiotics can mean losing the ability to walk unassisted.

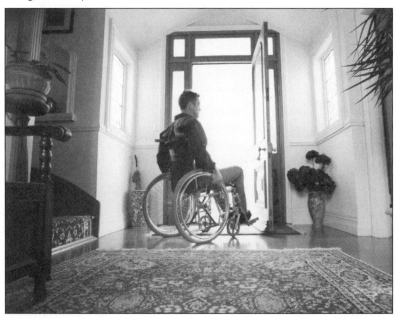

oral antibiotics, but is suffering from depression and guilt, feeling she is to blame for her parents' debilitated condition."[61]

Overreported?

Many people like Kevin and his family who are struggling with the disease and its costs hoped that the more the general public was aware of the problems faced by Lyme disease patients, the greater the chance of correcting them. However, they are meeting resistance within the medical community—doctors who believe that far too much media attention has been paid to Lyme disease. They say that the countless articles about how common the disease is, and how dangerous it can be, are misleading.

Many doctors have questioned the large number of people being diagnosed with Lyme disease—especially in the chronic stage. Many have psychiatric symptoms, such as clinical depression, confusion, and panic attacks, along with the more typical Lyme symptoms such as joint pain. One doctor pointed out that while some memory loss can occur in ongoing Lyme infections, such cases are quite rare.

Another doctor agreed, saying that patients are eager to have an answer to their health problems, and a diagnosis of chronic Lyme provides that—even when it is an incorrect diagnosis. "They'd rather have Lyme disease than multiple sclerosis, which has no cure," he said. "They'd rather have Lyme disease than depression, which carries a stigma. They'd rather have Lyme disease than something that nobody can figure out."[62]

Misgivings

One doctor who believes strongly that Lyme disease is being overdiagnosed is Allen Steere, the physician who took an interest in Polly Murray's case back in the 1970s. Steere was responsible for pushing researchers to find the cause of the disease. And while he was one of the first to realize that if untreated, Lyme disease could lead to ongoing health problems, Steere has recently had misgivings.

He has spoken out against the thousands of cases of chronic Lyme disease that are being diagnosed and has insisted that the scientific evidence does not support the large numbers of people who are being treated for months—and years—on end with antibiotics. Reading a letter from a woman complaining of mood swings, sleep problems, allergies, dizzy spells, and a host of other symptoms, Steere felt that she had been diagnosed in error. "What I suspect is that she doesn't have Lyme disease," he said, "but some kind of psychiatric illness. That doesn't mean that I don't care about her," he adds, "or what happens to her."[63] However, he insisted that putting such patients on many months' worth of antibiotics would not be helping them at all.

Steere has repeated what some other doctors have said— that long-term regimens of antibiotics can actually harm a patient, doing damage to the digestive system, bone marrow, and liver. In addition, they say, long-term use can make certain types of bacteria in the body resistant to the drugs. This means that in the future, when that patient needs antibiotics for a case of strep throat, for example, the antibiotic would no longer be effective.

A Major Controversy

Not surprisingly, Steere and those who agree with him have touched off a major controversy. There are many doctors who adamantly disagree and say that instead of being overdiagnosed, Lyme disease is still underdiagnosed in the United States. They say that there are thousands—perhaps tens of thousands—who have Lyme disease but have been diagnosed with some other health problem. As a result, such patients are not getting the help they need.

New York doctor Joseph Burrascano is one of the most vocal critics of Steere and his colleagues. He maintains that there are many cases of chronic Lyme disease, where for some reason or other the Bb bacteria resists the antibiotics and causes any number of strange symptoms. "Patients come to us after Steere and his colleagues deem them treated and cured," Burrascano said, "and we are able to demonstrate clearly, through biopsies and cultures and DNA probes, that they were still infected."[64]

However, Steere maintains that there are other explanations for the ongoing symptoms. One of the most likely, he says, is that some of these patients suffer from tissue and organ damage sustained while they had Lyme disease. Even though the disease itself was knocked out by antibiotics, the damage lives on—and will not be cured, no matter how many antibiotics are prescribed, or for how long.

"Steer Clear of Steere!"

Those who have been diagnosed with ongoing or chronic Lyme disease have been anything but silent observers of the controversy. For them it is not simply a medical difference of opinion, it is a red-hot political issue. Many patients have met with so much resistance getting doctors to test them for Lyme disease that they have formed patient advocacy groups. Other patients have used the Internet, finding support from others with similar stories.

These patients, together with some of the doctors who have diagnosed them, have become harsh critics of Steere, who they say has become a threat to Lyme patients everywhere. They believe that they have become as sick as they are because of arrogance and ignorance on the part of the medical establishment. And,

The Internet gives Lyme disease patients the opportunity to contact others with similar problems, seek out information regarding their illness, and form advocacy groups.

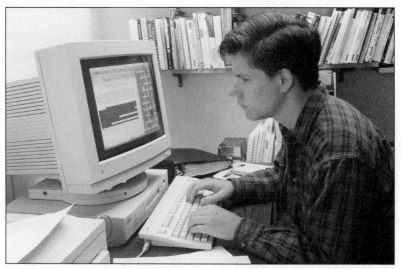

they say, because of Steere's reputation as a pioneer of Lyme disease, his doubts about chronic Lyme disease are being taken very seriously by other doctors as well as insurance companies that decide on guidelines for payment of medical claims. If Steere and other researchers are convinced that a few weeks of antibiotics are enough to cure Lyme disease, say advocacy groups, insurance companies that often pay for months of treatment will cut back. And that, they say, may have all sorts of ill effects on their health.

Wearing green ribbons, the symbol of what is called "Lyme solidarity," many of the patients turn out for meetings or hearings where health policies relating to Lyme disease are being discussed, or where dollars for medical research are being allocated. Some stand, some are in wheelchairs or lean on canes. They hold signs emblazoned with slogans like "Ticked Off!" and "Steer Clear of Steere!"

"We Are in Real Turmoil"

The medical issue is long from settled, say experts, since there is convincing evidence for both sides. However, it worries many Lyme patients that if scientists such as Steere feel that chronic Lyme disease is rare, millions of dollars that should be going for Lyme research may be derailed. Patients who have struggled for so long to find a doctor who would take them seriously worry that those doctors might be prevented from treating them with antibiotics for long periods of time if guidelines are adopted.

Karen Vanderhoof-Forschner, whose son died of chronic Lyme disease and who went on to start the Lyme Disease Foundation, has been a vocal critic of Steere and his research doubting the prevalence of chronic Lyme disease. Polly Murray, who says that Steere is doing to patients what the medical establishment in Lyme, Connecticut, once did to her, has turned against Steere, too.

But beginning in 2001, guidelines advocating only limited use of antibiotics were adopted. In fact, in New York, where more cases of Lyme disease have been diagnosed than in any other state, doctors willing to prescribe long-term treatment are being investigated by the state licensing board. Calling such actions "witch hunts," Lyme advocates say that it is no wonder that the number of "Lyme-literate" doctors is shrinking.

That worries everyone—especially patients, who say they resent being treated as though they are imagining symptoms. "Thousands and thousands of us stay with these doctors because they are making us well," said one patient. "If they weren't, why would we put ourselves through the physical and financial costs?"[65]

Another woman just shakes her head. "We are in real turmoil," she sighs. "If someone had told our doctors to stop [treatment after three or four weeks], some of us wouldn't be here."[66]

Despite the controversy, scientists continue Lyme disease research and seek more accurate tests that can tell whether someone has Lyme even in the early stages. Researchers also study the DNA of the Lyme bacterium to find a more effective cure. They hope to find a solution that will cure patients regardless of which stage of the disease they suffer from.

Chapter 7

Avoiding Lyme Disease

While there are obviously two very different ideas about the nature of chronic Lyme disease, there is something on which every patient, doctor, or researcher would agree—that avoiding Lyme disease entirely is far preferable to being sick with it. Since Willy Burgdorfer isolated the bacterium that causes the disease, researchers have worked on a vaccine that would prevent people from getting Lyme disease. By being vaccinated, people would not need to worry about avoiding ticks.

Despite spending over two decades searching for a preventive Lyme disease vaccine, science still remains unable to provide one.

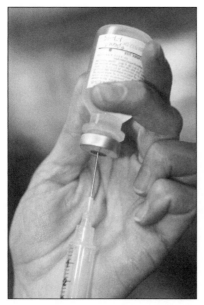

A Short-Lived Vaccine

In the mid-1990s, it seemed as if such a vaccine was a very real possibility. It was tested on hundreds of volunteers around the United States. But while some of the test subjects experienced no ill effects from the vaccine, other reported serious health problems. Edward Schneider, a New York resident who is an avid gardener, was eager to try the vaccine. Because he lives in an area that has a lot of Lyme disease, he knew that he was at risk for getting it, too.

But six weeks after getting his second dose of the vaccine, he experienced some paralysis, fever, and painful arthritis-like pain. "I would just like to know what the heck I have," said Schneider soon afterward, "because I always have been very healthy."[67]

Others have experienced the same problems, and some experts believe that one of the proteins contained in the drug can trigger a disease called autoimmune arthritis, a painful, degenerative condition that is untreatable. They believe that some people's cells have certain genetic structures that are vulnerable to the drug's protein, and people with that particular genetic makeup are at risk. The drug's makers disagreed; they claimed that they had tested the vaccine for such problems and had found none. The Food and Drug Administration monitored the testing and agreed that the vaccine was safe. Most likely, the ill effects experienced by some of the trial subjects were not related to the vaccine, they said.

However, after the vaccine was put on the market there continued to be people who showed symptoms of autoimmune arthritis, as well as other complaints. Such cases made many people reluctant to be vaccinated, and sale of the drug decreased quickly. By early 2002, the company pulled the drug off the market.

With no vaccine for Lyme disease available, it seems that people must look to other methods to prevent infection. Unfortunately, while there are some things that people can do to minimize their risk of Lyme disease, it is still maddeningly easy to become infected with it.

Not Easy to Avoid Ticks

When the research on Lyme disease was in its early stages, scientists were fairly sure that that risk was limited to the areas of the United States that had a sizable deer tick population—New Jersey, New York, Connecticut, Rhode Island, Massachusetts, Wisconsin, and Minnesota. In the mid-1980s, researchers acknowledged that there were a small number of cases in a few

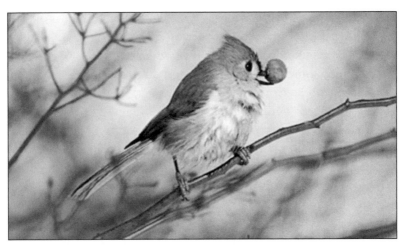

Ninety-nine different bird species within the United States are known carriers of deer ticks, dropping ticks that may have Bb each time they land.

other states, but more than 90 percent of the cases occurred in the previously mentioned seven states.

The list grew as years went by, however, and in 2002 scientists say that forty-nine states have reported cases of Lyme disease—only Montana has no reported cases yet on federal records. Even so, experts say that the higher incidence of the disease is creeping inland from the East and West coasts, and even into Canada. The reason for the spread of Lyme disease is simply that the deer ticks themselves are far more common than they once were.

Scientists know now that they travel not only on deer and mice, but on at least ninety-nine different species of birds—some of which are infested with hundreds of the ticks. As the birds stop to rest and feed, they are believed to pass infected ticks along the way. Dogs and people can carry ticks from one setting to another without knowing it.

New York City?

Many people still believe that it is primarily campers and other outdoor types of people who get Lyme disease, but that is not so. To avoid ticks, a person would also need to avoid golf courses, backyards, and gardens, for plenty of people have been bitten by ticks in those settings, too.

There have been cases of people being infected almost everywhere—including the heart of New York City. Denise Chapman, an emergency medical worker, was infested with a number of ticks and lice as she attended to an injured homeless person in an ambulance. Though she had removed the pests from her body after her shift was over, she found several embedded ticks the next morning. Within a few weeks, she had signs of Lyme disease, which has become an ongoing problem for her. Although Chapman's case was rare, it serves as a reminder that anything that looks like a tick should be examined closely, and removed quickly, say experts.

Taking Precautions

Understanding the growing prevalence of deer ticks as well as the varied settings in which they can be found is a good first step, say experts. One who is vacationing or is new to an area should contact a local natural resources official to ask whether Lyme disease has been a problem in the area. If so, it is important to know how to take precautions when outside—especially when walking in wooded areas, fields, or anywhere that grass is long.

Posted warning signs near trails should be noted with extreme caution when the presence of Lyme disease-toting deer ticks is likely.

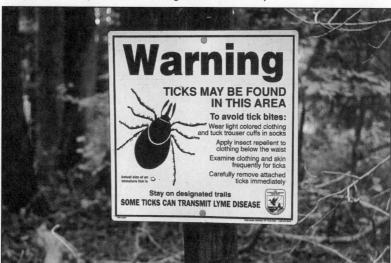

An insect and tick repellent is recommended for people who are spending time outside. Experts say that the most effective repellents contain a chemical known as DEET, which was developed originally for U.S. troops during the 1950s. DEET is especially effective against ticks and is so strong that it is not necessary to use a lot of it. Doctors also urge users to apply such repellent only in a well-ventilated area, since the fumes can be harmful.

There are important things to remember when dressing for the outdoors, too. Wearing white or light clothing helps, for ticks are more easily visible on light colors. A long-sleeved shirt and a pair of jeans will protect bare skin on arms and legs. People who are gardening are advised to use wide masking tape or duct tape to secure the cuffs of their shirt to their skin, so ticks cannot get underneath to bare skin.

Wearing light colors, long-sleeved shirts, thick pants, socks, and closed shoes can protect people from tick bites in high-risk areas.

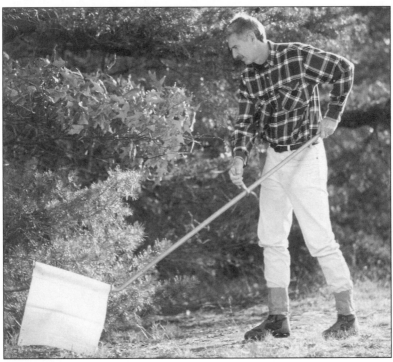

Shoes that tie are better than loose slip-ons or sandals. "Wear socks, too," says Chelsea. "I learned that from a brochure the doctor gave me after I was diagnosed. You're supposed to tuck your pant legs into your socks—that way the ticks can't sneak in under the bottom of your pants and crawl up your legs."[68]

After Being Outside

After coming inside, a shower is a good way to rinse off any ticks that may be crawling in hair or on skin. Afterward, it is important for people to check themselves thoroughly for ticks. Hard-to-see places are especially inviting for ticks—between toes, in the waistband area of underwear, and in groin and underarm areas, too. Clothing that has been worn outside can be put in the dryer for fifteen minutes at high temperature. The heat will kill any ticks that are on the clothes.

When one finds a tick, it is important to remove it carefully. If it is not yet attached to the skin, it can be removed with the fingers. However, doctors warn, it is not a good idea to squeeze or crush a tick with one's fingernails, for doing so may release germs from inside the tick.

Ticks that are already attached are a bit more difficult to remove, because they insert their barbed mouth parts deeply into the skin. Blunt-tip, fine-point tweezers are best for the job; tweezers with sharp points can puncture the tick and cause it to release its germs, along with the blood it has already fed on. Grasping the tick with tweezers as close to the skin as possible, and without twisting the tick's body, one should simply pull the tick straight back, using steady pressure, say doctors.

Often the mouth parts may remain in the skin after the tick's body is removed. Doctors recommend using a sterilized needle to remove them just as one would remove a splinter from under the skin. Afterward, a person should apply some antibacterial ointment and make sure hands are washed thoroughly.

Disposing of Ticks

One can burn an unattached tick after removing it. Another method involves tape, as explained by one Lyme expert: "Make a tape-tick sandwich by carefully sticking a generous piece of tape over the tick. Lift the tape with the tick still attached and fold it over. Voilà a tick sandwich. Be sure to discard it outside your home."[69]

A tick that was attached can be examined by a medical laboratory to see if it is carrying Bb bacteria. It needs to be alive for the bacteria to be seen, so it is important to put it in a tightly-sealed plastic bag or a pill container with a little piece of moistened cotton or tissue. A tick can stay alive in such a container for four or five days. Any local or state health department has a list of laboratories that will do free tick tests.

Discouraging Ticks and Their Hosts

Besides learning to find, remove, and destroy ticks that may appear on their clothing or skin, some people have found ways to cut down on the number of ticks living in their vicinity. For instance, some who live in rural areas have bought flocks of guinea hens—fat, short birds that thrive on eating hundreds of ticks each day. Others have trimmed vegetation on their property and have been conscientious about keeping grass cut short.

"We took down twenty trees on my parents' property up north," says one Wisconsin man. "That was hard, because those trees really added character to the place. My mom especially was against cutting them down. But those trees added a heck of a lot of shade—and ticks really like the shade. My dad has already had Lyme twice, and even though he recovered quickly with the antibiotics, he didn't want to go through that again."[70]

It is also possible to eliminate ticks by discouraging the animals that host them. In some areas, people have suggested that hunting regulations be relaxed so that hunters may kill more deer, which carry ticks. However, experts have found that the tick population is affected very little by this. A 1994 study in New York found that even with the reduction of a deer herd by 70 percent, there was no significant drop in the tick population. Ticks simply find other hosts, such as mice.

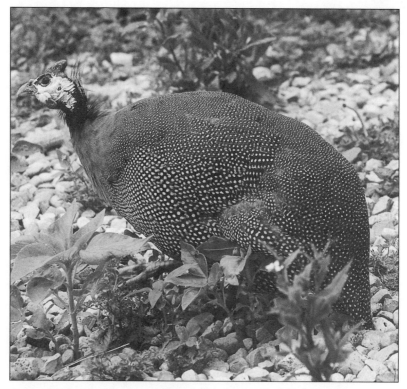

Guinea fowl (pictured) eat hundreds of ticks each day, helping to keep the yard of a rural home Lyme disease-free.

"Make Them Listen to You"

Most Lyme disease experts stress that the most important aspect of prevention is knowledge. If people understand the symptoms of Lyme disease, as well as the dangers of deer ticks, they can be more involved in their own health. "It's not smart to leave everything to doctors," said one Lyme disease sufferer. "Some of them are very knowledgeable, but others haven't seen much Lyme disease. So they don't always recognize the symptoms. Why take a chance that you'll get the doctor that doesn't know?"[71]

Joe, who had recently had Lyme disease, agreed. "People need to take charge of their case, I think. Be proactive. If you suspect you might have Lyme disease, demand a test. Make them listen to you."[72]

Experts say that it is a mistake to minimize Lyme disease as a minor problem. One doctor, who had also had Lyme disease, explained, "This is the kind of disease which, if not recognized and treated promptly and completely, can affect the future of our country. I have seen active, outgoing people end up in wheelchairs without the proper treatment. . . . This is scary stuff. And when you think that more than 50 percent of those infected with Lyme disease are teenagers and kids, we're talking about a real impact on our future."[73]

Notes

Introduction: The Faces of Lyme Disease

1. Personal interview, Chelsea, September 2, 2002, Brooklyn Park, MN.
2. Ray Glier, "Simpson Rejoins PGA Tour After Fighting Lyme Disease," *USA Today*, February 5, 1997, p. 14C.
3. Glier, "Simpson Rejoins PGA Tour," p. 14C.
4. Quoted in Glier, "Simpson Rejoins PGA Tour," p. 14C.
5. Personal interview, "David," September 30, 2002, Minneapolis, MN.
6. Telephone interview, John, October 4, 2002.
7. Telephone interview, Cherie, October 8, 2002.

Chapter 1: The Sickness Without a Name

8. Polly Murray, *The Widening Circle: A Lyme Disease Pioneer Tells Her Story*. New York: St. Martin's Press, 1996, p. 12.
9. Murray, *The Widening Circle*, p. 28.
10. Quoted in Murray, *The Widening Circle*, p. 58.
11. Murray, *The Widening Circle*, p. 4.
12. Murray, *The Widening Circle*, p. 86.
13. Quoted in Murray, *The Widening Circle*, pp. 118–19.
14. Alan G. Barbour, *Lyme Disease: The Cause, the Cure, the Controversy*. Baltimore: Johns Hopkins University Press, 1996, p. 28.
15. Murray, *The Widening Circle*, p. 12.
16. Quoted in Karen Vanderhoof-Forschner, *Everything You Need to Know About Lyme Disease and Other Tick-Borne Disorders*. New York: John Wiley & Sons, 1997, p. 38.

Chapter 2: From Deer Tick to Human

17. Susan Carol Hauser, *Outwitting Ticks*. New York: Lyons Press, 2001, p. 2.

18. Quoted in Vanderhoof-Forschner, *Everything You Need to Know About Lyme Disease*, p. 20.

19. Telephone interview, Marnie, September 30, 2002.

20. Telephone interview, Kyle, October 2, 2002.

21. Barbour, *Lyme Disease*, p. 61.

22. Telephone interview, Steve, September 13, 2002.

Chapter 3: The Signs of Lyme Disease

23. Telephone interview, Steve, September 13, 2002.

24. Personal interview, Laura, October 8, 2002, Richfield, MN.

25. Telephone interview, Cherie, October 8, 2002.

26. Barbour, *Lyme Disease*, p. 14.

27. Telephone interview, Joe, October 8, 2002.

28. Telephone interview, John, September 20, 2002.

29. Personal interview, Rich, September 24, 2002, Minneapolis, MN.

30. Telephone interview, Joe, October 8, 2002.

31. Hilary McDonald, "Lyme Disease Is More Than a Tick Bite," Personal Stories of Lyme Disease, May 1996. www.geocities.com.

32. Quoted in Barbara Wickens, "A Life of Pain," *Macleans*, February 6, 1989, p. 54C.

33. Murray, *The Widening Circle*, pp. 111–12.

Chapter 4: Diagnosis and Treatment

34. Barbour, *Lyme Disease*, p. 78.

35. Telephone interview, Joe, October 8, 2002.

36. Telephone interview, Cherie, October 8, 2002.

37. Denise Lang, *Coping with Lyme Disease: A Practical Guide to Dealing with Diagnosis and Treatment*. New York: Henry Holt, 1997, p. 51.

38. Personal interview, Raymond, September 14, 2002, Minneapolis, MN.

39. Personal interview, Rich, September 24, 2002.

40. Barbour, *Lyme Disease*, p. 123.

41. Personal interview, Rich, September 24, 2002.

Chapter 5: The Most Serious Lyme Disease

42. Vanderhoof-Forschner, *Everything You Need to Know About Lyme Disease*, p. xi.

43. Quoted in Wickens, "A Life of Pain," p. 54.

44. Quoted in Nora Underwood, "A Growing Menace: Doctors Debate the Spread of Lyme Disease," *Maclean's*, September 10, 1990, p. 37.

45. Personal interview, "David," September 30, 2002.

46. Quoted in Lang, *Coping with Lyme Disease*, pp. 103–4.

47. Telephone interview, Kathleen, August 28, 2002.

48. Quoted in Lang, *Coping with Lyme Disease*, p. 171.

49. Lyme Alliance, "Lisa I's Story," Lyme Quilt Page. www.angelfire.com.

50. Lyme Alliance, "Cynthia's Story," Lyme Quilt Page. www.angelfire.com.

51. Personal interview, "David," September 30, 2002.

52. Lyme Alliance, "Rafelle's Story," Lyme Quilt Page. www.angelfire.com.

Chapter 6: Beyond the Symptoms

53. Quoted in Lang, *Coping with Lyme Disease*, p. 15.

54. Marie Ciasullo, "Faces of Lyme Disease," Lyme Disease Foundation. www.lyme.org.

55. Personal interview, "David," September 30, 2002.

56. Personal interview, "David," September 30, 2002.

57. Lyme Alliance, "Mary H's Story," Lyme Quilt Page. www.angelfire.com.

58. Quoted in Jane Gross, "In Lyme Disease Debate, Some Patients Feel Lost," *New York Times*, July 7, 2001, p. B1.

59. Lyme Alliance, "Tim's Story," Lyme Quilt Page. www.angelfire.com.

60. Telephone interview, Kathleen, August 28, 2002.

61. Lang, *Coping with Lyme Disease*, pp. 192–93.

62. Quoted in David Grann, "Stalking Dr. Steere," *New York Times Magazine*, June 17, 2001, p. 6.

63. Quoted in Grann, "Stalking Dr. Steere," p. 6.

64. Quoted in Grann, "Stalking Dr. Steere," p. 6.

65. Quoted in Gross, "In Lyme Disease Debate, Some Patients Feel Lost," p. B1.

66. Quoted in Gross, "In Lyme Disease Debate, Some Patients Feel Lost," p. B1.

Chapter 7: Avoiding Lyme Disease

67. Quoted in Ephrat Livni, "Vaccine Victims?" ABC News.com, May 17, 2000. www.abcnews.go.com.
68. Personal interview, Chelsea, September 2, 2002.
69. Vanderhoof-Forschner, *Everything You Need to Know About Lyme Disease*, p. 119.
70. Telephone interview, Paul, October 15, 2002.
71. Telephone interview, Paul, October 15, 2002.
72. Telephone interview, Joe, October 8, 2002.
73. Quoted in Lang, *Coping with Lyme Disease*, p. 28.

For Further Reading

Books

James N. Parker and Phillip M. Parker, eds., *The 2002 Official Patient's SourceBook on Lyme Disease*. San Diego: ICON Health Publications, 2002. The most up-to-date information, with good sections on clinical trials and works in progress on new types of prevention.

Daniel Rahn and Janine Evans, eds., *Lyme Disease*. Philadelphia: American College of Physicians, 1998. Technical, but good section on the management of Stage I Lyme disease.

Scott Veggeberg, *Lyme Disease*. Springfield, NJ: Enslow Publishing, 1998. Very readable; helpful section on the overdiagnosis of Lyme disease.

Periodicals

Marlene Cimons, "Lyme Aid," *Runner's World*, June 2001.

Frederic Golden, "The Ticks Are Back: And Thanks to El Niño, There May Be More Than Ever," *Time*, June 8, 1998.

Christine Gorman, "Tick, Tick, Tick . . . ," *Time*, July 28, 1997.

Sandra Levy, "Lyme Disease Prevention: Here's What to Tell Patients," *Drug Topics*, March 20, 2000.

Paul Raeburn, "A Genome Project Against Disease," *Business Week*, July 1, 2002.

Internet Sources

Lyme Alliance, Alan Saly, "Denise C's Story," Lyme Quilt Page. www.angelfire.com.

Lyme Alliance, "Stories of Chronic Lyme Disease," Lyme Disease Quilt Page. www.angelfire.com.

Lyme Disease Foundation, "Faces of Lyme Disease." www. lyme.org.

Organizations to Contact

American Lyme Disease Foundation
Mill Pond Offices
293 Route 100
Somers, NY 10589
(914) 277-6970
www.aldf.com
This organization supports research and works to provide reliable and scientifically accurate information to the public and the health care provider.

Centers for Disease Control and Prevention (CDC)
Atlanta, GA 30333
(404) 639-3311
www.cdc.gov
The CDC is a federal agency whose mission is to develop and apply disease prevention and control, environmental health, and health promotion and education activities designed to improve the health of the people of the United States.

The Lyme Alliance
PO Box 454
Concord, MI 49237
www.lymealliance.org
The Lyme Alliance is an international organization that provides information, support, and advocacy for victims of Lyme disease and their caregivers. Its website offers personal stories of Lyme victims as prevention tips.

Lyme Disease Foundation (LDF)
One Financial Plaza, 18th Floor
Hartford, CT 06103
800-886-LYME
www.lyme.org
The Lyme Disease Foundation is a nonprofit medical health care agency that is dedicated to finding solutions to tick-borne disorders. The LDF believes that in order to find real solutions, four key groups must work together—the public, scientists, government, and private businesses. It maintains a website with a great deal of current medical and political information.

Works Consulted

Books

Alan G. Barbour, *Lyme Disease: The Cause, the Cure, the Controversy.* Baltimore: Johns Hopkins University Press, 1996. Somewhat difficult reading, but good detail on the types of antibiotics that are used to cure Lyme disease.

Susan Carol Hauser, *Outwitting Ticks.* New York: Lyons Press, 2001. Brief but very clear information on the deer tick and its life cycle.

Denise Lang, *Coping with Lyme Disease: A Practical Guide to Dealing with Diagnosis and Treatment.* New York: Henry Holt, 1997. Very helpful information on the political aspects of Lyme disease.

Polly Murray, *The Widening Circle: A Lyme Disease Pioneer Tells Her Story.* New York: St. Martin's Press, 1996. Fascinating first-person account of Murray and her family's health problems. Very readable.

Karen Vanderhoof-Forschner, *Everything You Need to Know About Lyme Disease and Other Tick-Borne Disorders.* New York: John Wiley & Sons, 1997. Excellent bibliography and very comprehensive index.

Periodicals

Ray Glier, "Simpson Rejoins PGA Tour After Fighting Lyme Disease," *USA Today,* February 5, 1997.

David Grann, "Stalking Dr. Steere," *New York Times Magazine,* June 17, 2001.

Jane Gross, "In Lyme Disease Debate, Some Patients Feel Lost," *New York Times,* July 7, 2001.

Nora Underwood, "A Growing Menace: Doctors Debate the Spread of Lyme Disease," *Maclean's,* September 10, 1990.

Barbara Wickens, "A Life of Pain," *Maclean's*, February 6, 1989.

Internet Sources
Ephrat Livni, "Vaccine Victims?" ABCNews.com.
Lyme Alliance, "Cynthia's Story," Lyme Quilt Page. www.angelfire.com
———, "Lisa I's Story," Lyme Quilt Page. www.angelfire.com.
———, "Mary H's Story," Lyme Quilt Page. www.angelfire.com.
———, "Rafelle's Story," Lyme Quilt Page. www.angelfire.com.
———, "Tim's Story," Lyme Quilt Page. www.angelfire.com.
Lyme Disease Foundation, Marie Ciasullo, "Faces of Lyme Disease." www.lyme.org.
Hilary McDonald, "Lyme Disease Is More Than a Tick Bite," Personal Stories of Lyme Disease. www.geocities.com.

Index

Picture Credits

Cover photo: © Alfred Pasieka /SPL/Photo Researchers, Inc.
Courtesy of American Lyme Disease Foundation, Inc., 41
Courtesy of ARS/USDA, Scott Bauer, 9, 28, 31
Courtesy of ARS/USDA, Keith Weller, 76
© Scott Bartel/SPL/Photo Researchers, Inc., 50
© Olivia Baumgartner/CORBIS SYGMA, 59
© Scott Camazine/Photo Researchers, Inc., 20
Courtesy of Centers for Disease Control, 21
© Custom Medical Stock Photo, 14, 23, 44
© E.R. Degginger/Photo Researchers, Inc., 30
Jeff DiMatteo, 27, 38
Courtesy of Centers for Disease Control/PHIL/Jim Gathany, 26
© Gilbert S. Grant/SPL/Photo Researchers, Inc., 75
© David M. Grossman/Photo Researchers, Inc., 55
© Eunice Harris/Photo Researchers, Inc., 17
John Radcliffe Hospital/SPL/Photo Researchers, Inc., 35, 39
© LWA – Stephen Welstead/CORBIS, 42
© Doug Martin/Photo Researchers, Inc., 64
© Carolyn A. McKeone/SPL/Photo Researchers, Inc., 79
© Jose Luis Pelaez/CORBIS, 53, 62
© M. Peres/Custom Medical Stock Photo, 32, 48
PhotoDisc, 19, 25, 56, 58, 69, 72, 74
© Michael Pole/CORBIS, 66
© Pete Saloutos/CORBIS, 46
© Tom Stewart/CORBIS, 45
© Larry Williams/CORBIS, 65

About the Author

Gail B. Stewart received her undergraduate degree from Gustavus Adolphus College in St. Peter, Minnesota. She did her graduate work in English, linguistics, and curriculum study at the College of St. Thomas and the University of Minnesota. She taught English and reading for more than ten years.

She has written over ninety books for young people, including a series for Lucent Books called The Other America. She has written many books on historical topics such as World War I and the Warsaw ghetto.

Stewart and her husband live in Minneapolis with their three sons, Ted, Elliot, and Flynn; two dogs; and a cat. When she is not writing, she enjoys reading, walking, and watching her sons play soccer.